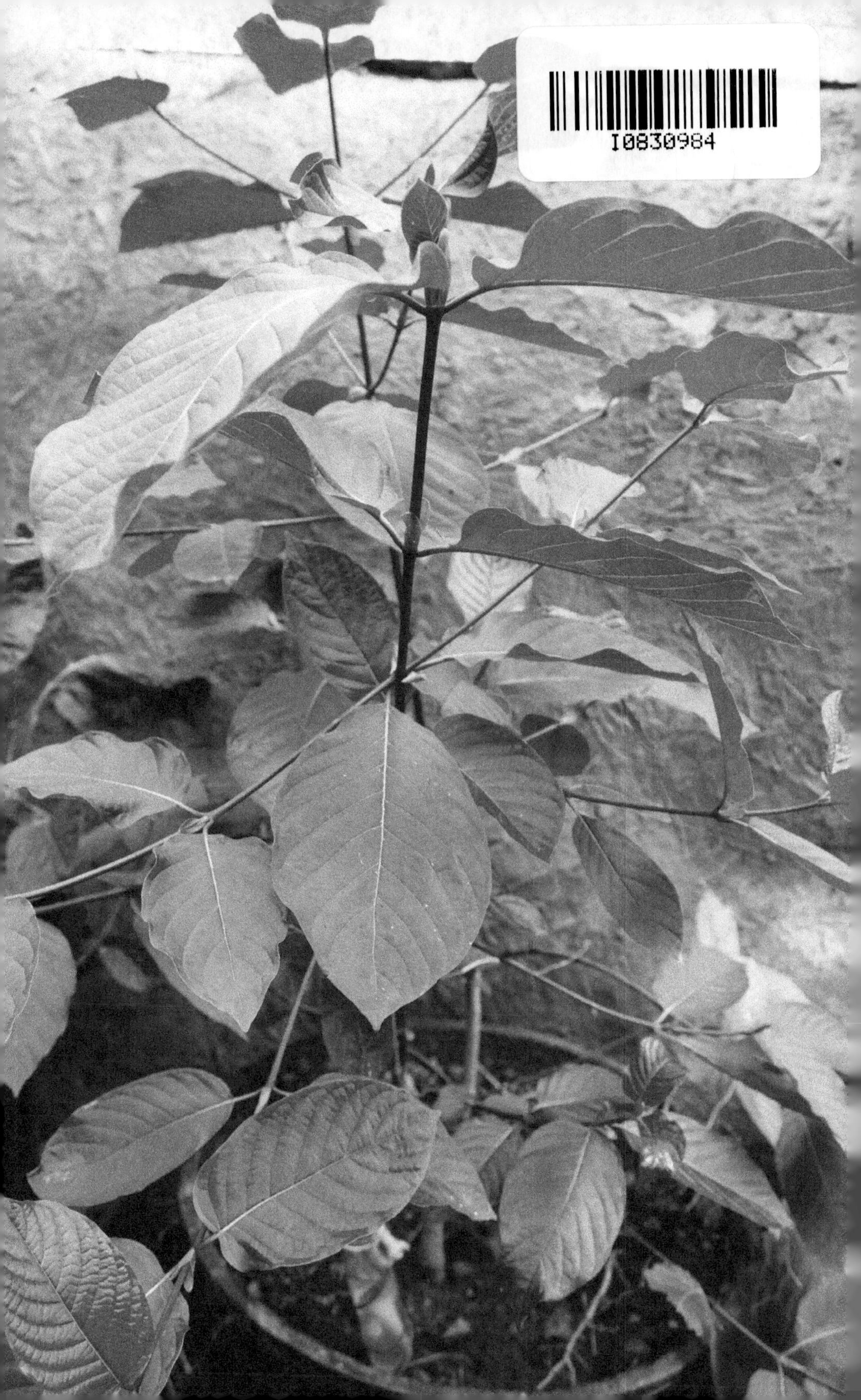

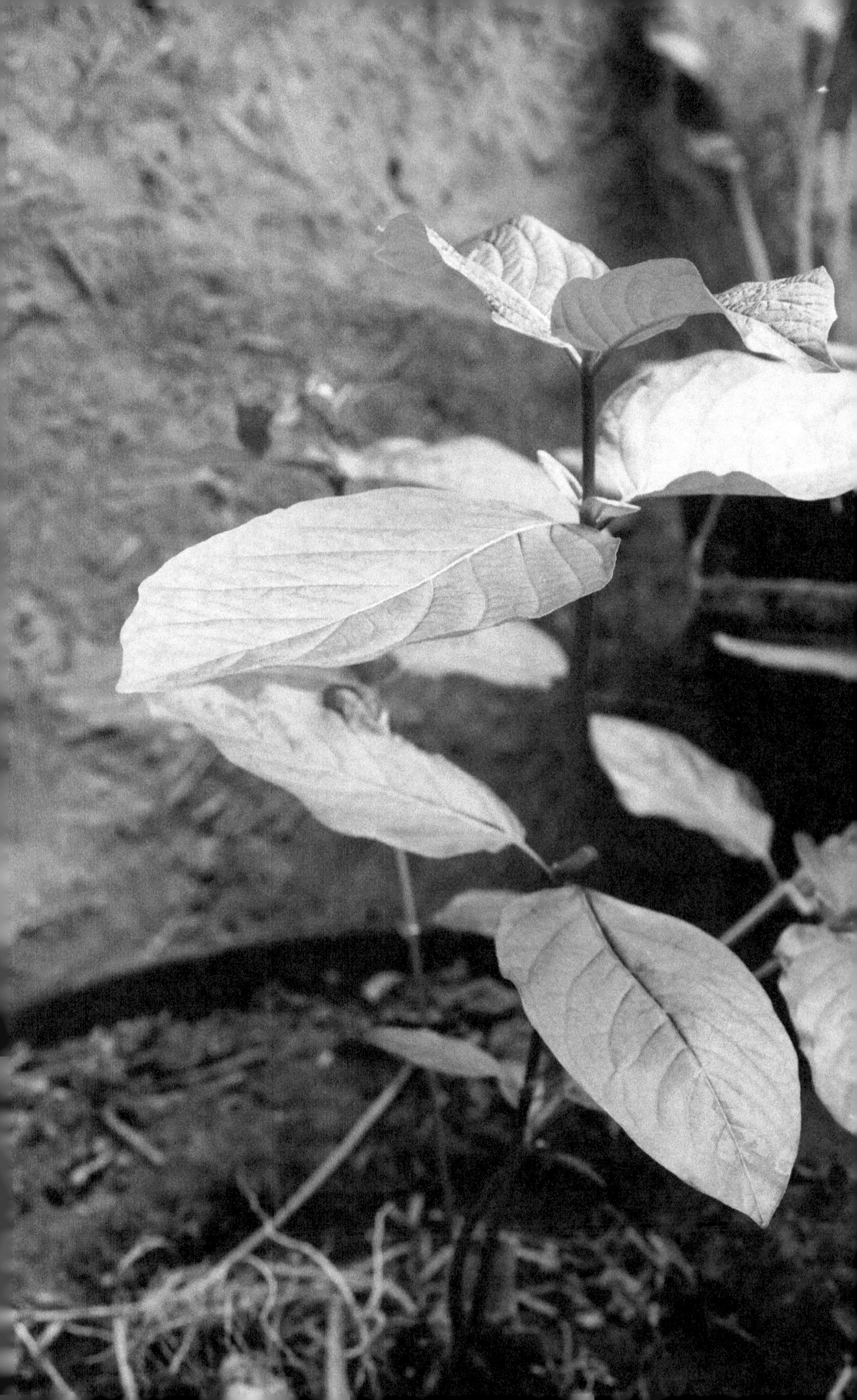

KRATOM

THINGS YOU NEED TO KNOW TO USE IT SAFELY

By **Dan Chiras & Linda Stuart-Chiras**

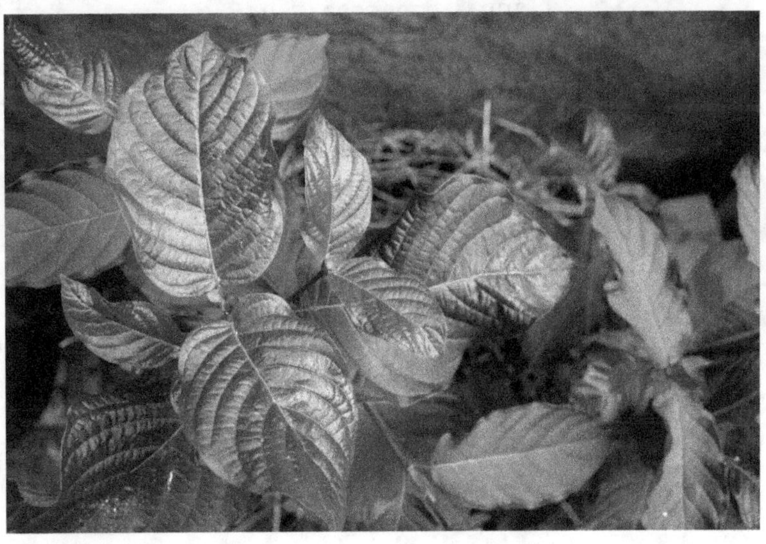

Design and Layout by Riley O'Laughlin
Co-owner of You Select Created, a graphic design, marketing, and photography company

CATALOGING IN PUBLICATION DATA:

A catalog record for this publication is available from the National Library of Congress

Copyright © 2021 by Daniel D. Chiras and Linda Stuart-Chiras
All Rights Reserved

Cover Design and layout by Riley O'Laughlin

Printed in the United States by Sustainable Systems Design
First Printing, December 2020

ISBN: 9798552247486

Inquiries regarding requests to reprint all or part of this book should be addressed to Dan Chiras at the address listed below,

Sustainable Systems Design, Inc.
3028 Pin Oak Road
Gerald, MO 63037-1212
(636) 303-9884

To order a copy e-mail Dan Chiras at
danchiras@evergreeninstitute.org

✎ DISCLAIMER ✎

This book is for informational purposes only. We present information that is accurate to the best of our knowledge. Although we point out why Kratom is used – and has been used historically -- and its purported benefits, we do not offer medical advice. Your physical and mental health are unique and require careful consideration on your part. We do offer advice to proceed cautiously, consult with a medical professional if you have any questions about other medications you are taking, and learn as much as you can. You may also want to seek counsel of a trusted medical doctor or naturopathic doctor or another healthcare professional who you can trust – and one who is open to alternative medicine. Always purchase Kratom from highly trusted sources.

We highly recommend that you research Kratom, including dosages, safety, and addiction potential prior to using this herbal medicine. The American Kratom Society's (AKA) website contains a plethora of information, including links to scientific papers on health benefits and several other important topics. We were initially told to check out the Botanical Education Alliance and United Kratom Association. It appears, however, as if these organizations have merged with AKA or are sharing the same website, speciosa.org.

It's definitely worth reading the "negative" coverage of Kratom on the WebMD and the Mayo Clinic websites, too. That way you can make up your own mind.

We do not make claims of the benefits of Kratom, except those that we've personally experienced – and even then, remember that what we experience may not be relevant to you. Bear in mind that our experience is somewhat limited and the effects we report may be different than those you experience.

In this book, we disclose information we've gleaned from books and other publications by people with considerable experience using Kratom. That said, we emphasize that no warranties of any kind are declared or implied in this book.

Be sure to consult regulations in your state, county and city to be sure that purchase and use are legal. I've listed cities, counties, states, and countries where Kratom use is illegal or regulated, but remember that rules change. To stay abreast of changes in legal status, be sure to consult resources like the American Kratom Association. It keeps track of Kratom's legal status throughout the United States.

We reiterate: we are not rendering legal, financial, medical, psychological or any other professional advice. Your needs are individual, and we can't pretend to make recommendations for you.

Always remember that different people react differently to the same medication and dose of any medication. So, proceed carefully.

Please note that various authors recommend that you start with low doses and that you do not take Kratom with other drugs or medicines, including alcohol, opioids, or any type of stimulant. Virtually all our resources suggest that you switch strains often to avoid the possibility of dependency or addiction. Numerous authors warn against using concentrated Kratom or products made from concentrates, as you may have no warranty of their contents. Dried leaves and powder derived from them, say most authors, are the safest choices, provided you are purchasing them from a reputable source.

The reader acknowledges and agrees that under no circumstance are the authors responsible for any losses, direct or indirect, that may result from the use of information presented in this book, including errors, omissions, or inaccuracies.

A WORD OF CAUTION

Kratom is sold in the United States as a dietary supplement. Here are a few things you should know about dietary supplements before using Kratom:

• Federal laws in the United States do not require supplement makers to prove that their products are safe before marketing them to consumers.

• Dietary supplements may have more or less of an ingredient than the label claims — which means you could end up taking way more *or way less* than you had intended. If you buy from unscrupulous sellers, *you may end up taking none at all. (Italics mine)*

• Dietary supplements aren't intended to treat or cure disease. Using a supplement together with medicines or in place of a prescribed medicine could harm your health.

Source: Kratom: A Look at the Risks and Possible Side Effects Related to Taking the Herbal Product. Published online in Everyday Health. Written by Lindsey Konkel. Medically reviewed by Robert Jasmer, MD.

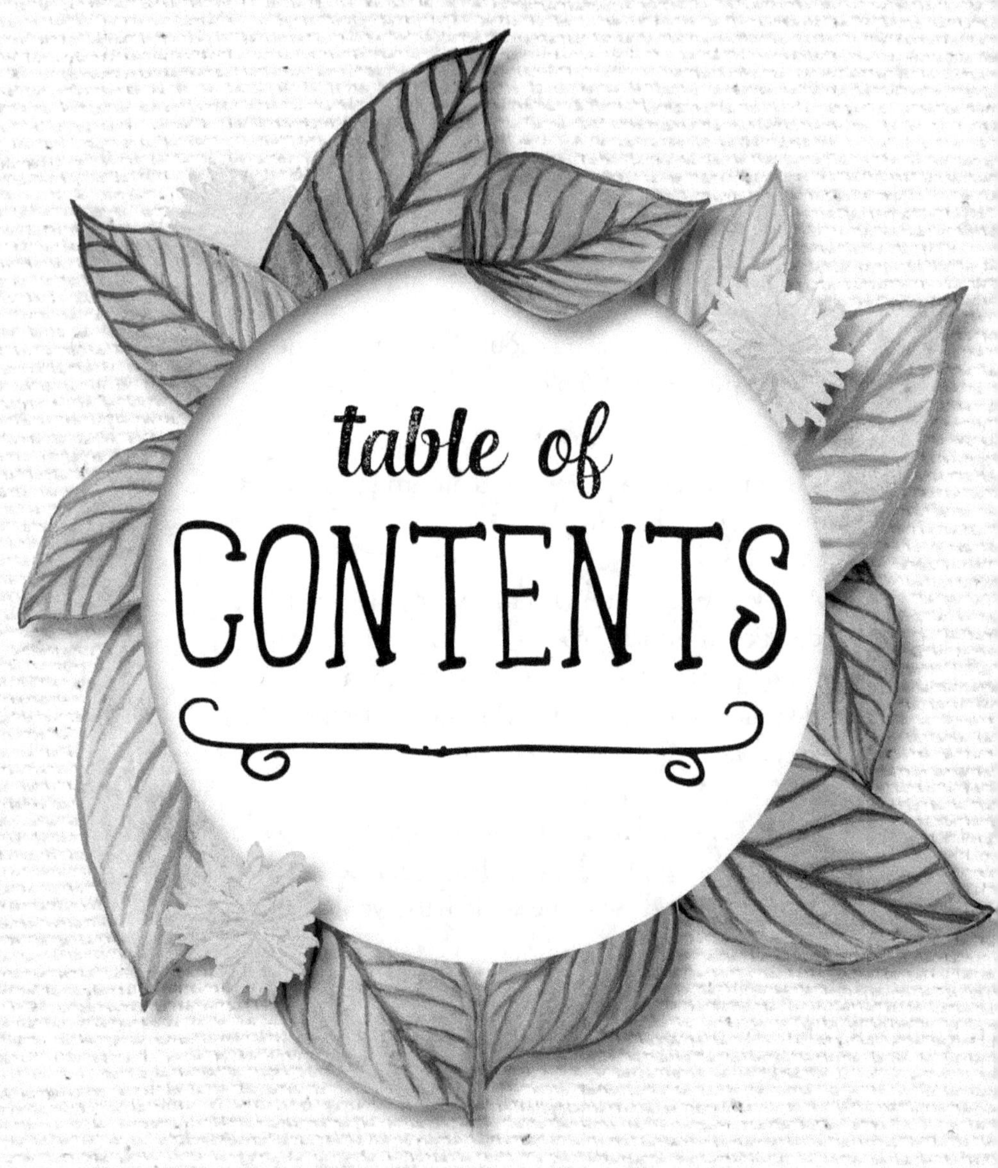

table of
CONTENTS

01

OUR INTRODUCTION TO KRATOM

Linda started using Kratom in 2019 to relieve intense pain resulting from two badly worn-out knees, damaged by many years of jogging in some pretty difficult terrain – the foothills of the Rocky Mountains in Colorado.

We visited an orthopedic surgeon who said that she'd lost a lot of cartilage in her knees and was "bone on bone" in both knees. Unfortunately, the surgeon refused to operate, proclaiming in his Godlike manner that she "was too young." (She was 55 at the time).

His recommended course of action was to inject steroids every three to four months in both knees to relieve the swelling and pain. He said he'd surgically replace the knees when Linda could no longer walk. Sounds like sound medical advice, eh? It's like, don't get this car fixed until the axle breaks. Drive it until you crash, then we'll fix it.

We didn't think the advice made a whole lot of sense but trusting our doctor (like idiots) we complied. Linda started receiving steroid injections. This course of treatment persisted for three years, and guess what? It worked. The steroids reduced swelling and made life tolerable. She could walk without pain. In addition, she noticed that pain in other parts of her body like her hip and shoulder decreased after each steroid injection. Stupidly, we counted this as a blessing. It was clear that the steroids were leaking into her bloodstream, providing widespread relief from pain. What a bonus!

After a year or so, Linda started losing hair and bruising and experiencing extreme skin thinning. She not only lost virtually all her body fat; she lost a considerable amount of muscle. Her arms and legs became sticks. Over a couple years of steroid injections, her weight plummeted from 125 to 90 pounds.

Severe bruising occurred as a result of inconsequential bumps into solid objects on the farm. Her arms and legs turned black and blue, and her skin started to tear with the slightest scratch or abrasion. Her forearms became a roadmap of scars. Her mental status went to hell, too. She became extremely anxious, irrational, depressed, and wildly emotional. Making matters worse, she also became extremely forgetful. She lived in a mental fog.

Assured by the orthopedic surgeon that the steroids couldn't be to blame for Linda's symptoms -- because "steroids don't leave the joint capsule of the knee" – Linda and I spent a couple years visiting our primary care physician and specialists to try to figure out what was wrong with her. These doctors ran many tests and examined numerous possibilities. Unfortunately, the tests revealed that there was nothing wrong with her. All the while, her mental and physical health continued to deteriorate. At one point, we both got to thinking that she was dying.

At the very first visit Dan suggested that Linda was displaying symptoms that looked a lot like adrenal insufficiency. Three years late, our primary care physician agreed to a test for this disease: an adrenal stress test. She ran the test and guess what: Linda's adrenal glands were not performing well. At that point, we were referred to an endocrinologist, an internal medicine doctor who specializes in hormone disorders. This was three years after our initial visit.

After examining Linda and running some more tests, he concluded that the steroids she'd been receiving were indeed leaking into her bloodstream, shutting down her adrenal glands. Linda was suffering adrenal insufficiency caused by steroids. Three years of steroid injections most likely led to Linda's massive weight loss, thinning skin, bruising, a host of other symptoms like her memory issues and anxiety.

Six months after the endocrinologist advised that she discontinue steroid shots, her skin began to thicken and the skin tearing, bruising, and bleeding greatly diminished. She also came out of the steroid cloud.

One problem solved.

Bolstered by this development, we visited her orthopedic surgeon. He agreed that it was time to replace her knees. However, because her skin had thinned so much he could not to operate on her. Why?

There was not enough dermis in her skin to suture the incision. Her skin was like crepe paper. (The dermis is a layer of connective tissue under the most superficial layer of skin, the epidermis.) Although Linda needed surgery badly, she had to wait until the dermis grew back a bit -- if it could. Who knew how long that would take?

There was another problem, however. Being off steroids placed Linda in incredible pain. Her knees were bone on bone, as noted earlier, and the grinding of bones on bone hurt like hell. Going up and down stairs or hilly terrain was not only painful but extremely difficult.

The issue we faced while waiting for her skin to regenerate was how to kill the pain so Linda could carry on some semblance of a normal life. Traditional over-the-counter pain killers did nothing to relieve the pain. CBD oil didn't seem to do much to help either. Rather than take opioid pain killers, Linda started taking Kratom powder.

Much to our surprise, she found that it helped – not just a little but a lot. It allowed her to function without the mind-numbing pain. It was still difficult to navigate inclines or declines and stairs, but she could move about without the excruciating pain.

Bolstered by her success, Dan started using Kratom to relieve stress and knee and foot pain caused by a mild case of arthritis. He found it extremely helpful.

Spurred on by our initial success, we decided to research Kratom use. What we discovered was a minefield of conflicting information. Opponents of Kratom, like the FDA, claimed that it has little, if any, medicinal value and, to make matters worse, is addictive.

Proponents offer an entirely different view. To them, Kratom is a wonder herb.

So, what's the truth?

Is Kratom a medically beneficial herbal medicine that's safe to take or is it ineffective and potentially addictive?

That's the principal question we sought to answer in our research. This book is an attempt to present the best and most accurate information we could find so readers like yourself can make up your own minds. We also decided to provide a considerable amount of background information about Kratom, so you can fully understand what it is and, if you choose to use it, how to use it safely. Let's start with the basics.

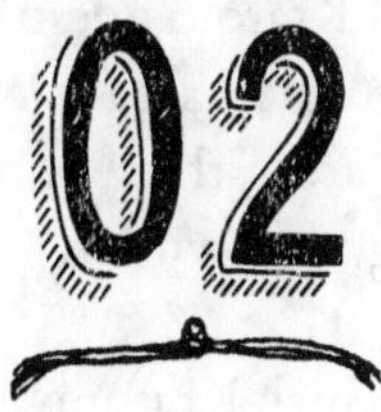

KRATOM BASICS

How is Kratom pronounced?

American's commonly pronounce Kratom with a hard "a" with emphasis on the first syllable: KRAY-tem. Think crayfish.

The correct pronunciation is with a soft "a" and emphasis on the second syllable, kruh-TOM. The U in Kruh sounds like in "crush."

Needless to say, you can pronounce it any way you like. It sounds less harsh when pronounced correctly. It's more exotic too, much like the countries it comes from. Softening the word may also soften people's perceptions of this plant and it's purported medicinal benefits.

What is Kratom?

Kratom is a substance derived from the leaves of trees that grow wild in Southeast Asia. Although the Kratom tree is an evergreen, it's not like a pine, fir, or spruce tree with sharp pointed wax-coated needles. Rather, Kratom has wide green leaves like many deciduous tree species growing in North America and Europe. It just doesn't shed them, hence its classification as an evergreen. Kratom doesn't lose its leaves because it occupies subtropical and tropical areas blessed with warm humid weather year-round. In such areas, there's no need to shed its leaves and go dormant to endure a long, cold winter.

Interestingly, the tree from which Kratom herbal remedies are derived is a member of the coffee family. (For those who must know, it's a member of the Rubiacaea family (pronounced rew-be-A-see-I). It's scientific name is *Mitragyna speciosa*. That's pronounced my-trah-GUY-nah spee-sea-OH-sa.

The Rubiacaea family is rather large group containing an estimated 13,000 species. Approximately 60 of the species, Kratom among them, are used in folk medicine to treat 70 diseases or medical conditions.

What does it's scientific name mean?

Mitragyna speciosa was so named because the primary chemical constituent, responsible for many of its reported health benefits, is a chemical known as mitragynine (pronounced my-trah-GUY-neen.)

Does Kratom have any other names?

Kratom goes by many different names in different parts of the world. Here are a few names it goes by in Thailand: ketum, kakum, thom, katuan, and thang.

Kratom goes by several other names in Thailand and other countries. In the Philippines, for instance, it is referred to as Mambog. In Vietnam, it's called Giam.

Where in Southeast Asia does it grow?

The simple answer to this question is "All over the place."
Kratom trees *(Mitrogyna speciosa)* are native to a handful of countries in and around Southeast Asia. We found it difficult to nail down

the list, but it appears as if Kratom is native to Indonesia, Thailand, Malaysia, Myanmar, Vietnam, and Papua New Guinea, and parts of the Philippines. It thrives in the warm temperatures of these countries and the moist soils found in them. It prefers soils with a pH of 5.5 to 6.5. (Keep that in mind if you decide to grow Kratom.)

One book we read claimed that Kratom also grows in Australia and New Zealand. We're assuming the tropical northern portions of these countries. We're not sure if it is native to these regions or simply grown in them because of favorable climatic conditions. We suspect that it's native to these regions.

> If your geographic knowledge of this part of the world is in need of a little help, it's a good idea to study a world map to locate the countries. Because many of you probably won't have a globe or world map at your disposal, I've attached these figures to help.

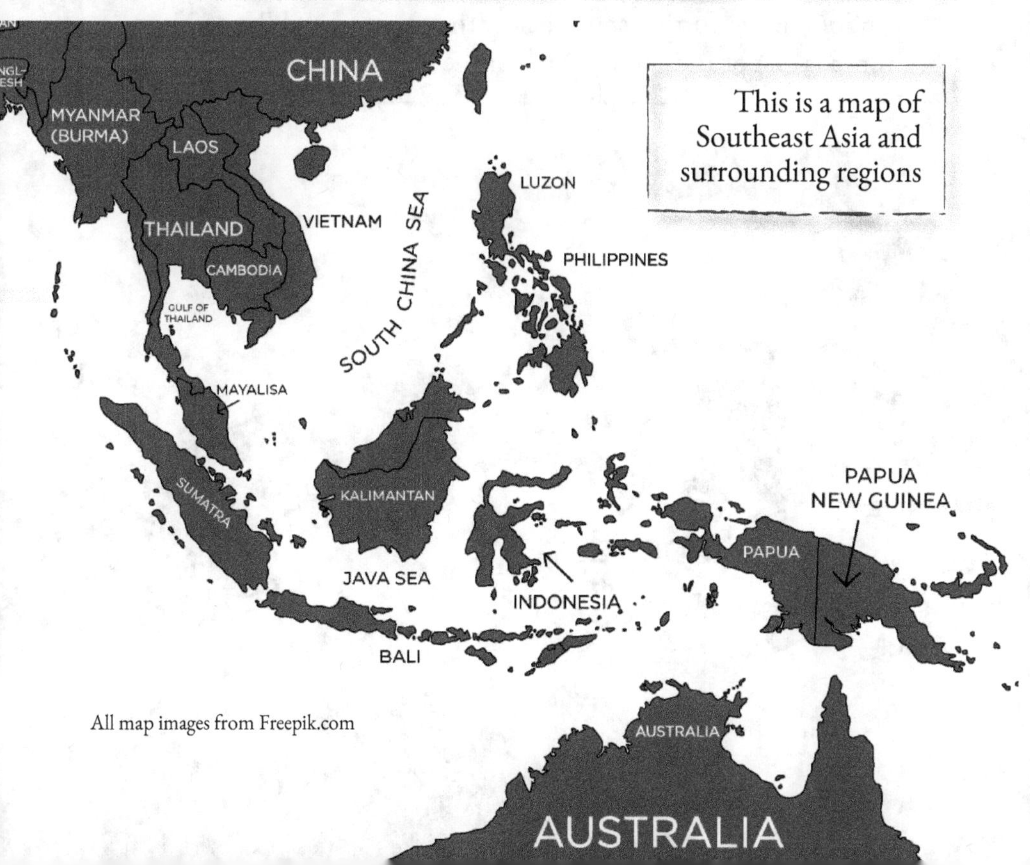

This is a map of Southeast Asia and surrounding regions

All map images from Freepik.com

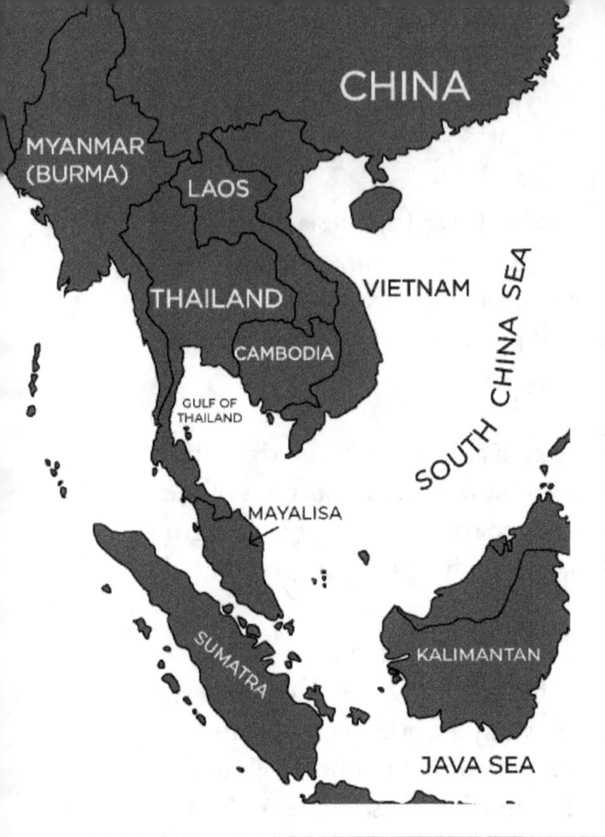

As shown in this figure, Southeast Asia is an oddly shaped piece of land attached to southern China. Vietnam is part of southeast Asia along with Laos, Cambodia, Myanmar and Thailand.

Malaysia lies below Southeast Asia.

Indonesia lies further south below the equator, and Papua New Guinea is east of Indonesia, north of the northeast part of Australia.

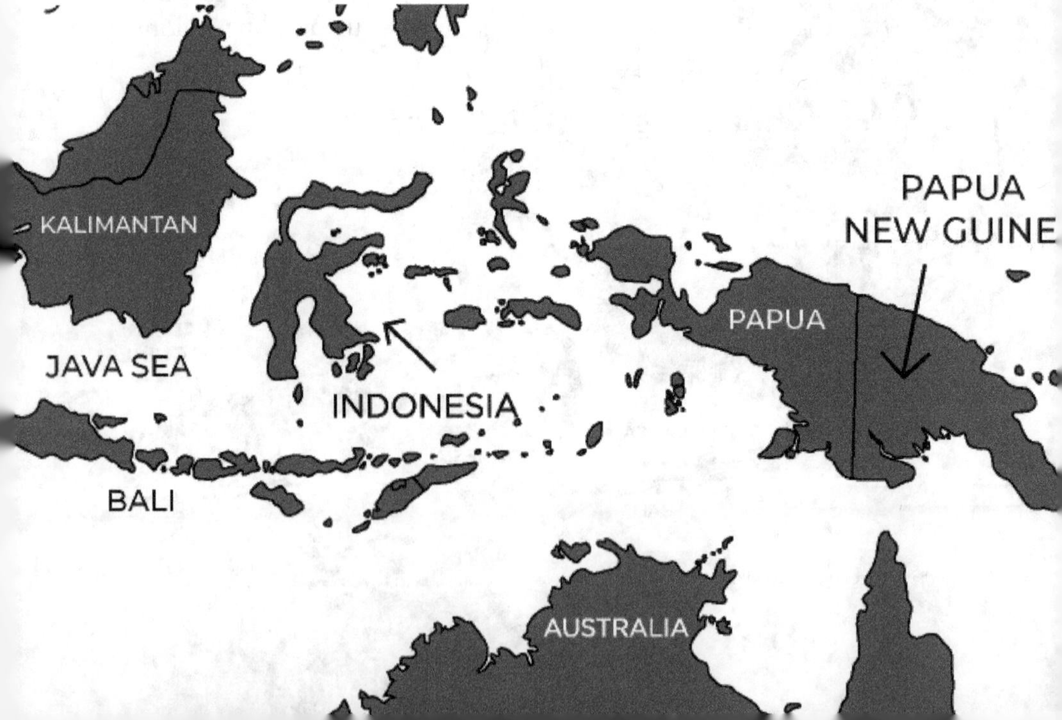

How tall does the Kratom tree grow?

Kratom is not a bush like coffee plants. It's a tree that grows quite tall. Some sources say it can achieve heights of 10 to 100 feet with a 15-foot diameter base, although 100-foot tall trees are reportedly rather rare. Most resources we've studied say it grows from 42 to 80 feet with trunks as big as 3-feet in diameter. The folks at Mytreesoflife.com say that most Kratom plants don't grow taller than 50 feet.

How tall it gets doesn't really matter.

The important point is that you can't grow Kratom in a greenhouse or in your living room unless you trim the sucker down and force it to grow more like a bush. Its height can also be curtailed by growing in a container such as a three-to-ten gallon pot. (More on growing Kratom later.)

When was it discovered by the Western World?

Mitragyna speciosa was first discovered in Thailand by a Dutch botanist, Pieter Willem Korthals. He described the tree in a publication in 1839.

When was Kratom Introduced in the United States?

Kratom was first introduced to the United States following the Vietnam War by Southeast Asia immigrants and returning soldiers. The latter had been introduced to Kratom during their service in Nam. These individuals continued its use to boost energy. (Some claim that the stimulatory effect of certain strains is similar to that from having a cup of coffee in the morning.) Kratom was also used by Vietnam veterans and immigrants to boost mood and combat pain. Immigrants acquired it either from friends and family members still living in Southeast Asia and from ethnic deli's that served these communities.

Where does it come from today?

While Kratom grows in many parts of Southeast Asia, it is imported principally from Indonesia.

It is also grown in the United States in semitropical regions like southern Florida. Still others grow Kratom indoors in their homes or apartments and in greenhouses where temperatures can be regulated. As noted earlier, it is a tropical plant and therefore prefers temperatures in the 70s and 80s. (More on this later.)

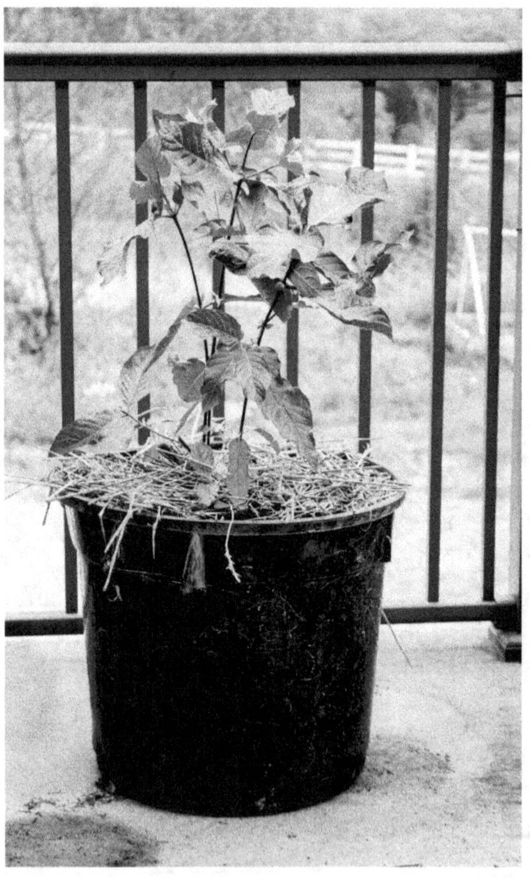

This small Kratom bush is growing on our patio. It thrived outdoors during our warm, humid summers and did well in the early fall. Now it's growing indoors in our passive-solar home. We placed it near a south-facing window where it gets plenty of sunlight.

POTENTIAL HEALTH BENEFITS

How Long has Kratom been used?

Kratom has been used in folk medicine for at least 200 years in Southeast Asia and neighboring countries—that is, by people without a doctor's prescription. As a result, Kratom is often referred to as a *naturally occurring plant medicine.*

Historically, why has Kratom been used?

Kratom has been used for a variety of reasons. Field workers in Southeast Asian countries, for instance, chewed the leaves to **increase energy levels**, in much the same way that natives of the Andes chewed coca leaves.

Kratom was also used to **relieve pain**. Workers found that it numbed aches and pains, and did so rather quickly. This helped workers feel better when engaged in tedious and physically demanding jobs.

Over the years, Kratom has also been used to **treat various ailments,** for example, to reduce fevers, manage diabetes, and treat diarrhea.

Kratom has also been successfully used to help heroin addicts break their addiction and ease withdrawal from this dangerous drug. In Southeast Asia, some addicts reportedly even switched to Kratom from heroin, finding it a much safer and less expensive. It's said that Kratom provides a similar sensation to opioids with much lower risk of addiction. We learned of a man in our town who had become addicted to opioids to kill back pain. He switched to Kratom and was able to kick his opioid habit painlessly.

How is Kratom used today?

Kratom is used today by tens of thousands of people to treat a wide assortment of ailments – sometimes under medical supervision, most times not.

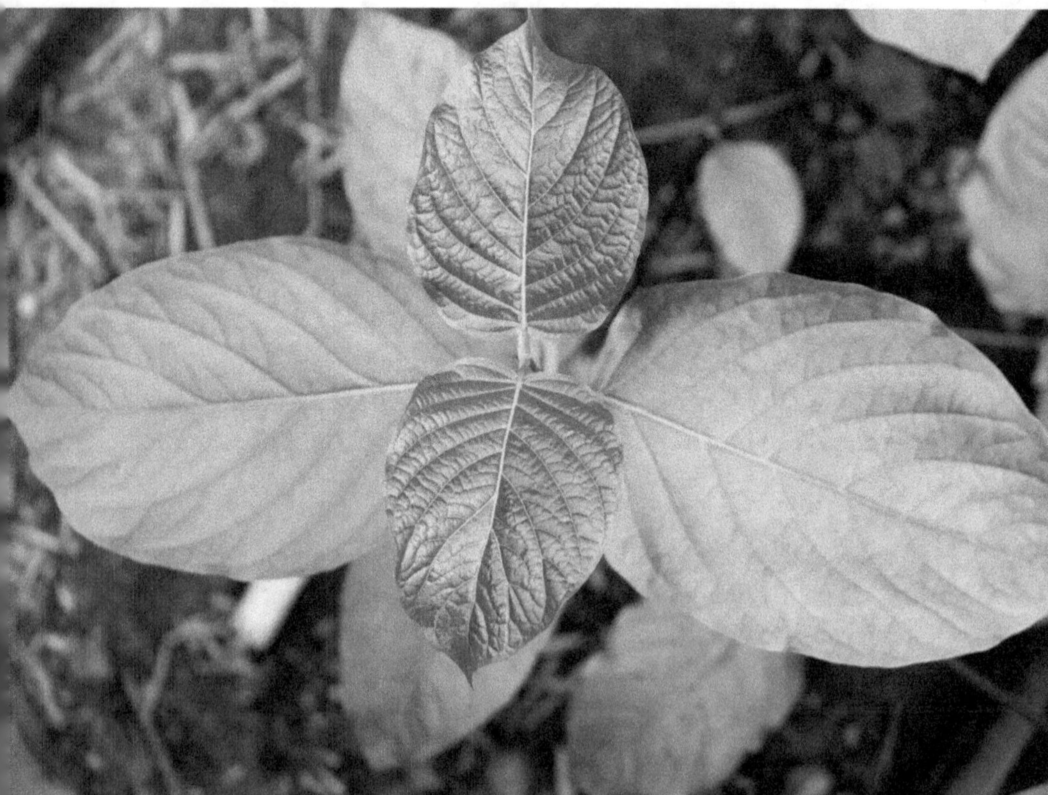

Some individuals take Kratom to combat Chronic Fatigue Syndrome. They report that it boosts their energy levels. Many college students take Kratom (specifically white-veined Kratom) to help them study longer and harder – no doubt cramming for tests. This strain of Kratom not only boosts energy, it also reportedly increases their ability to concentrate.

Pain relief is probably it's most sought-after benefit today. People suffering the chronic pain of arthritis constitute the largest users. We can personally confirm its analgesic effects, though our study only has "an n of two" – that's scientific lingo for saying there are only two subjects in our study.

Yet another common use of Kratom is to **relieve stress**. We've experienced that benefit as well. Dan finds that one type of Kratom (red-veined) helps him calm down (feel relaxed) when stressed or feeling jittery from too much caffeine.

Kratom also **elevates mood**. Many people agree that white- and green-veined Kratom have proven to be effective mood boosters. We both find that it gives us a sense of well-being – that all is well with the world – which isn't true, but it's nice to feel that way once in a while.

Many people take Kratom to **boost their immune systems**, making them better able to fight off potentially harmful viruses and bacteria and to ward off cancer. Others take Kratom because it contains antioxidants, naturally occurring chemical substances that neutralize potentially dangerous chemicals in our bodies known as free radicals. Free radicals are reactive chemicals that can cause cancer, hardening of the arteries, and, as medical scientists are now finding, a host of other diseases.

Kratom also reportedly helps reduce inflammation, which medical science is learning is at the root of a long list of diseases such as arthritis, heart disease, strokes, hardening of the arteries, diabetes, pancreatitis, asthma, and autoimmune diseases such a rheumatoid arthritis.

Kratom is used today to help wean folks from opioids such as heroin. As noted earlier, Kratom reportedly helps individuals free themselves from opioids without the hideous physical and mental side effects that typically accompany opioid withdrawal.

Some Kratom varieties – notably red-veined Kratoms – are used to **enhance sleep**, helping people who suffer from occasional or chronic insomnia. We've known several people who use it, in part, to achieve this goal.

As if these benefits aren't enough, some people claim that Kratom has an **aphrodisiac quality**. They even claim that it helps increase fertility, although both claims strike us as a stretch – perhaps a way to convert more people to users? Dan can say that Kratom makes him happier and more loving, but that's the extent of its "aphrodisiac benefits."

Here's a summary of Kratom's purported benefits:

- Relieves pain
- Increases energy levels
- Increases one's ability to concentrate
- Relieves stress and anxiety
- Elevates mood
- Boosts immune system
- Provides protection against diseases via its antioxidants
- Combats inflammation
- Combats fevers, manages diabetes, and treats diarrhea.
- Treats opioid addiction
- Helps patients detox -- quit opioid use without the harmful side effects
- Enhances sleep

NOT ALL KRATOM IS CREATED
EQUAL

As you shall soon see, Kratom's beneficial effects vary by the color of the veins in the leaves from which the powder is made.

Generally, Kratom made from red-veined leaves (RVK) are said to be more sedating. They deaden pain, provide calming effects, and enhance sleep. RVK is the powder that's used to treat opioid addiction.

In contrast. White-veined Kratom (WVK) leaf powders are said to be more stimulating. They increase concentration and boost energy.

The third type, green-vein Kratom (GVK) is said to offer both benefits. Its effects are in between
RVK and WVK.

All three varieties elevate mood and relieve pain.

What diseases is Kratom thought to be useful to treat or prevent today?

Kratom is used with and without prescription (usually without) by people all over the world to treat the following diseases, providing pain relief and possibly other benefits:

- Osteoarthritis
- Rheumatoid arthritis
- Fibromyalgia
- Cancer
- Multiple sclerosis
- Gallbladder disease
- Stomach ulcers

How effective it is, we can't say. There's not a lot of science behind the use of Kratom to treat medical disorders. Researchers throughout the world are working hard to gather data, but it is too early to tell.

Is Kratom used recreationally?

Why, of course.

When taking low-to-moderate doses, especially white and green-veined Kratom, people report feeling high -- that is, they experience a sense of euphoria – that all is well with the world. That's a rare and precious feeling these days.

Certain Kratom preparations are used because they make people feel happier, less self-conscious, and braver in social settings that evoke anxiety.

How can this herbal remedy have so many health benefits? Is that really possible?

I'm always skeptical when someone – whether it's a snake-oil salesman of the old West or a poorly informed herbal advocate – claims that a medication can successfully address a wide array of ailments. "This product will relieve migraines, shrink the prostate, improve memory, fight Alzheimer's, pay your taxes, reverse brain cancer, fight diabetes, wash your car, make your children behave, cause your skin to glow and your hair to shine, reverse aging, and boost sexual desire...among others."

Yeah, right.

In the case of Kratom, there's reason to believe that this herbal medicine could have many beneficial effects. Why?

First of all, Kratom contains a **large number of potentially beneficial chemical compounds.** To date, researchers have identified over **40**

chemical components, including 25 alkaloids, in Kratom.

Alkaloids are alkaline compounds (bases) produced by many plants. They often have profound effects on human physiology – some good, some not so good. This group of chemical compounds is rather large with wide-ranging effects.

Perhaps the best-known alkaloid is **nicotine,** a rather addictive stimulant produced by tobacco plants. It is ingested when tobacco is smoked or chewed.

The infamous pain killer **morphine** is also an alkaloid. It's highly addictive and is quite lethal when administered in high doses. When used by doctors in smaller amounts throughout the world, it is an excellent pain reliever.

Strychnine is another example of an alkaloid that's a poison in high doses. When I was growing up in western NY, I worked for a veterinarian. At the time, strychnine was used to euthanize dogs. They died a horrible death. Nowadays it is sometimes used today to kill "pests," such as birds and rodents.

Quinine is an alkaloid that's proved to be a valuable medicine. It was discovered in plants. Quinine has been synthesized in the lab and is now used to treat malaria. Hydroxyquinone is used to treat rheumatoid arthritis.

Atropine is an alkaloid used by physicians to treat pesticide poisonings. It also decreases salivary production during surgery, so you don't slobber all over the place. You'll find it in eye drops prescribed for certain diseases of the eye.

Kratom leaves produce a large variety of alkaloids—over two dozen. Some of them have been shown to lower blood pressure. Others block pain. Some increase blood flow in the brain, while others stimulate the immune system. Some chemical compounds are antioxidants that help prevent cancer. Some fight inflammation. This panoply of beneficial compounds found in Kratom could explain why it could legitimately be helpful in treating so many different ailments and provide such a wide array of benefits. But that's not all.

Not only are there are lot of different alkaloids in Kratom, some of them have multiple effects. Take for example, the main chemical component of Kratom, an alkaloid called ***mitragynine*** (MG).

Mitragynine stimulates certain nerve receptors (called adrenergic receptors) resulting in mild stimulation. But it also soothes coughing (it's an antitussive). It combats diarrhea and binds to certain receptor molecules on nerve cells that some opioids bind to, killing pain. And, as if that's not enough, MG also fights malaria much like quinine.

And as if that's not enough Kratom contains at least 15 other phytochemicals that provide medical benefits. (More on this shortly.)

> Notice the tiny whitefly on the leaf of this plant. Watch for this notorious insect pest. They can cause a lot of damage even in relatively small numbers. Also watch out for mealy bugs. Monitor indoor and greenhouse plants often and spray with insecticidal soap mixture to kill bugs.

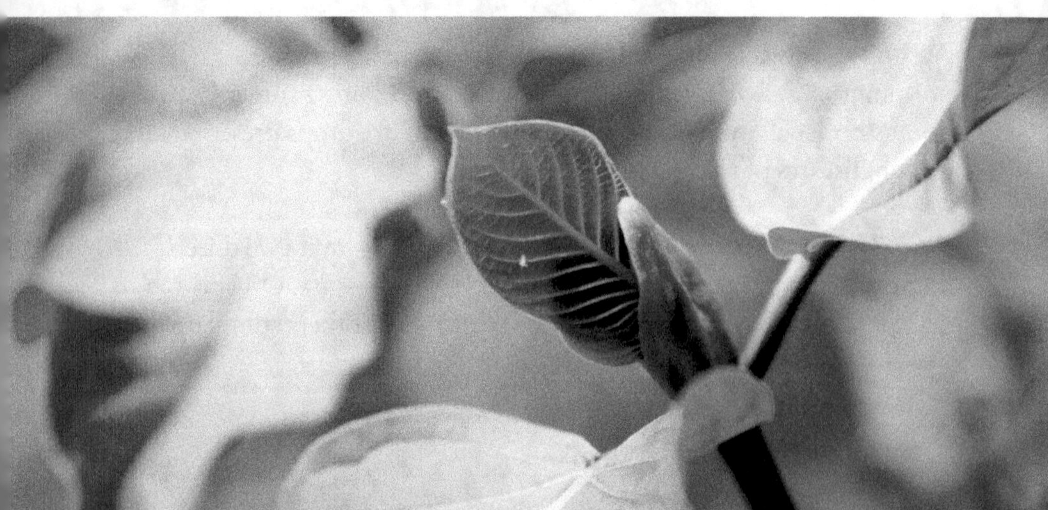

04

KRATOM VARIETIES AND THEIR POTENTIAL HEALTH BENEFITS

How do I know which Kratom to buy?

The **medical benefits you derive from Kratom vary with the strain** – notably whether the leaf comes from a species grown in Malaysia, Vietnam, or Indonesia, according to most sources. That's because trees from different regions contain different proportions of the active ingredients. That results in different effects.

The most significant difference in the medical benefits though, is probably due to the color of the veins in the leaves harvested from trees. Unbeknownst to many, all Kratom trees have leaves with three different color veins: red, white, and green. **Different vein-colored leaves contain different mixtures of alkaloids and other chemicals. That difference in chemical makeup results in different physiological effects.**

More on this shortly.

Okay, so how do I know what Kratom leaf color I should buy?

As a general rule, if you want sedative effects, that is to calm down and feel relaxed, take red-veined Kratom. If you want a boost of energy, take white.

If you want both, take a green-veined Kratom. Or, take yellow Kratom, which I'll explain later.

All three varieties elevate mood and relieve pain. They'll also provide antioxidant and anti-inflammatory benefits.

> Healthy leaves are deep green. They begin as a yellow green that deepens to a dark green, if plants are healthy (no bugs, proper pH soil and water).

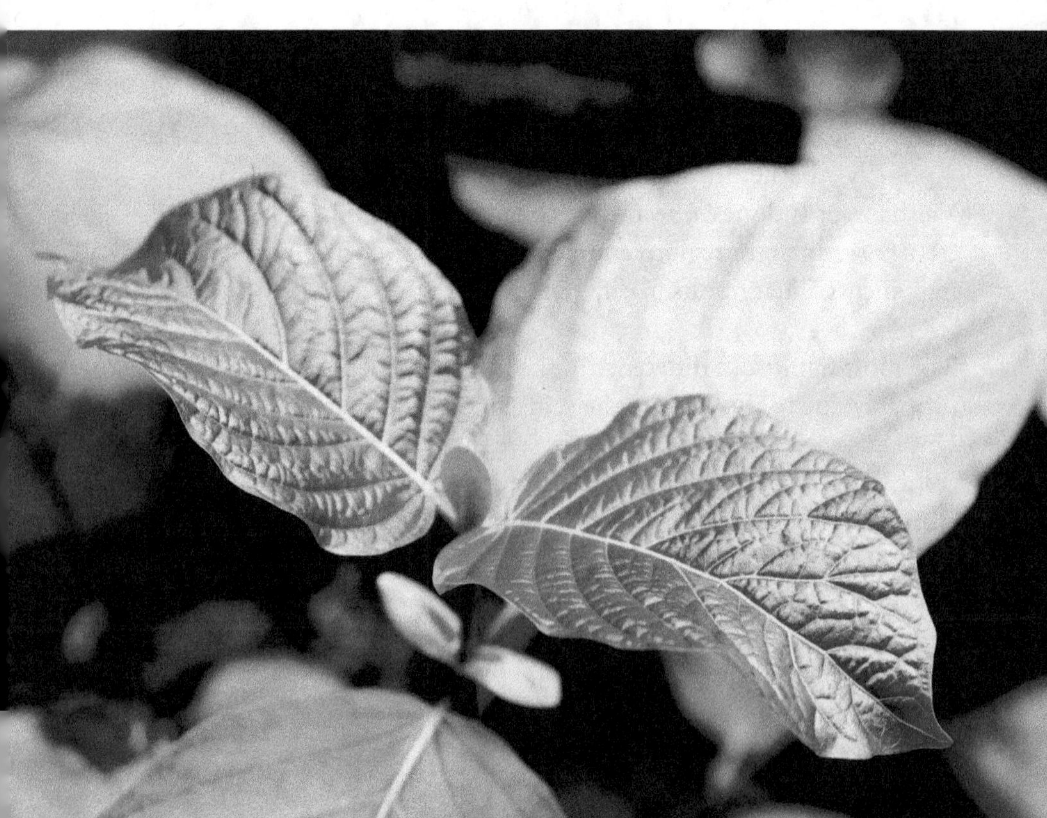

Can you help clarify the various strains I see advertised on the Internet?

Okay, you've done a little research on the Internet and you've read an article or two on Kratom. In your search for information, you've encountered vendors that advertise red-veined varieties of Kratom, for example, Red Indo or Red Borneo. They give buyers the impression that each of these is a "specific strain." In other words, Red Indonesia powder comes from an "Indonesian Kratom tree with red-veined leaves."

Unfortunately, that's not correct.

As noted earlier, all Kratom trees have leaves with all three vein colors. If a product is labeled Red Indonesian, it means it comes from red-veined leaves from a tree that is grown in Indonesia. Or, it could be red-veined leaves from a tree that originally comes from Indonesia but is now grown indoors in a greenhouse or outdoors in another country. Make sense?

All this is to say, Kratom products like capsules can be made from trees grown – in the wild or in cultivation – from different parts of the tree's range, for example, Borneo, Thailand, or Malaysia. So, if a seller says it a "Red Indo strain," it's from a tree grown in -- or originally from -- Indonesia. However, there is no such thing as a "Red Indo tree" – a tree that only produces red-veined leaves.

According to William Poole of mytreesoflife.com, these days nearly all Kratom comes from trees growing in the wild or on farms in Indonesia. Farmers often collect leaves from trees growing in different parts of the country. As they harvest leaves, they separate them by vein color. Manufacturers buy leaves with red, green, and white veins, then make their products. So, a "red-veined Indo strain" product is one made from red-veined leaves from a tree or several trees from Indonesia. A "green-veined Indo strain" product is one made from green-veined leaves from a tree or many trees from Indonesia. (As a side note, most reds are actually the result of a special curing process, which brings out more of that "red" effect.")

Now that you have that straight, there's some more confusing information we'd like to help set straight. As you study Kratom products you will encounter two strains advertised as "Red Maeng Da" and "Bali." However, there is no Red Maeng Da strain or Bali strains of the Kratom tree. According to Poole, the Indonesian have recipes that blend two or more leaf types to create special blends like Maeng Da and Bali.

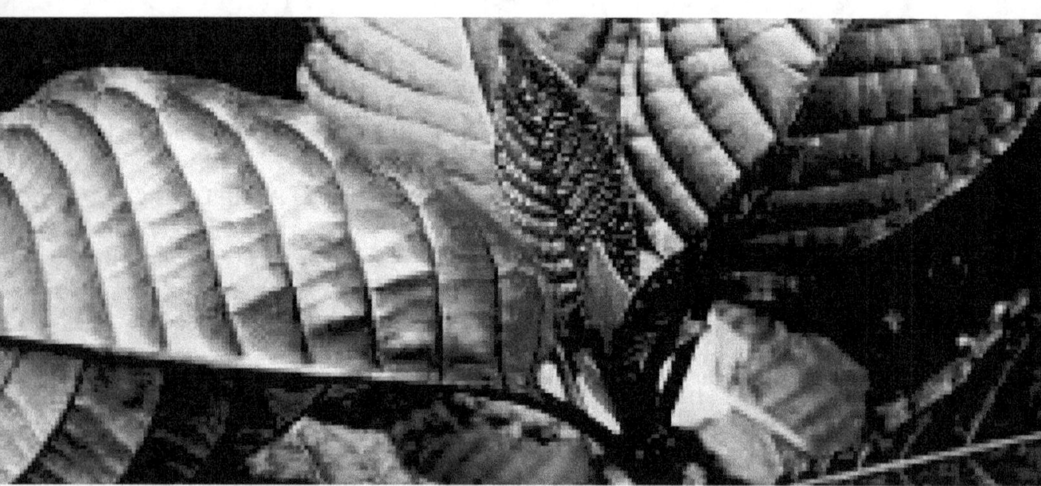

What does red-veined Kratom do?

If you're just starting out, most authors recommend you begin with red-veined Kratom. It's the most popular product.

That's because, RVK has **rather pleasant, soothing effects**. Mentally, most people report that red-veined Kratom (RVK) promotes an overall **sense of well-being and peace of mind**. In moderate doses, 3 to 5 grams, RVK makes a lot of people **feel optimistic.** All in all, RVK has a **pleasurable, calming effect.**

Unlike antidepressants that slowly lift you out of a glum mood, over a period of weeks and even months, RVK powder or capsules can make you feel happy almost immediately. We've found this to be true, but have noticed that RVK makes it bit more difficult for us to think clearly and remember things. Linda, for example, finds that RVK make it a bit more challenging to do math. She can't concentrate as well, either. I find that RVK calms me down, but I can't take it before musical performances. My performance really suffers when I have a little RVK coursing through my blood vessels. Sometimes I forget parts of songs that I know by heart.

Many sources say that RVK is also great for **promoting sleep**. You might give it a try. Those who report this effect, note that a moderate dose of RVK – around 5 to 10 grams of Kratom -- puts them to sleep rather quickly.

Physically, red-veined Kratom (RVK) **relieves pain**. What is more, when taken in lower dose RVK does so without making you drowsy, unlike many traditional and highly addictive pain meds. Therefore, RVK is often used by individuals and doctors in some parts of the world to **fight pain** caused by chronic conditions such as osteoarthritis, replacing highly addictive opiates.

As if that's not enough, RVK also seems to **relax muscles.**

Red-veined Kratom is also used to counter the horrid withdrawal symptoms of opioid (e.g., heroin) addiction, though the FDA argues that there's no conclusive proof of this benefit, even though it has been used in this manner for decades in Southeast Asia.

Bear in mind, there are differences in red-veined strains. RVK from plants grown in Thailand and Borneo, some say, have sedative effects, while red-veined leaves from plants grown in Sumatra result in an elevated or excited mood. Talk to others to get their opinions. Consult with online suppliers and try a couple to see which you like the best and how they affect you. It's a good idea to refrain from operating a vehicle or heavy equipment when taking RVK.

A FEW WORDS OF
CAUTION

Don't ever mix Kratom with alcohol, pain meds, or any dangerous drugs like cocaine, heroin, hydrocodone, Fentanyl, or other opioid pain medications.

Most authors recommend starting slowly, that is, taking two to three grams at first to assess the effects. If you're a tiny person, you may need to scale back a little. If you weigh more, you may want to try a slightly larger dose, but always be cautious.

To study your body's reaction to Kratom, try taking it at the same time of day and under the same conditions, for example, on an empty stomach. And take it the same way each time (e.g., by capsule) initially as you discover the effects it has on your body.

Take notes, and adjust dosages accordingly.

Remember also, that it takes time for Kratom's active ingredients to get into your bloodstream. So, don't rush things. How you take Kratom (capsule vs. powder) and whether or not you are taking it on an empty stomach will greatly affect its absorption. Even the time of day and your body weight may affect the time it takes to feel an effect.

What does white-veined Kratom do?

Unlike most RVK, white-veined Kratom or WVK is generally viewed as a **stimulant**. It's the most "energetic" Kratom. Here's why:

WVK, reportedly, **enhances alertness and concentration,** so it is often used by students who have put off studying to the last minute and need to stay awake and alert. Various authors recommend using it in low to moderate doses. Low being in the 3-to-5-gram range; moderate being in the 6-to-10-gram range. Remember, though, different people react differently, so be cautious.

WVK also generally creates **a bright, positive or cheery mood,** the kind of feeling you want when you're going out to meet new people or take on a new day.

At moderate to high doses, WVK creates a sense of euphoria. That feature also makes it popular among many individuals seeking to have a little fun.

In general, WVK is a pick-me-up.

Many people take it when they are feeling lethargic, wiped out, exhausted, sad, or depressed – or some combination of them. Some friends use it in the morning in place of a cup of coffee. That said, virtually every book or article we've read advises strongly against using any form of Kratom daily, for example, taking WVK as a daily energy boost. Bear in mind that there are other natural and healthy ways to boost energy: transitioning to a healthy lifestyle characterized by healthy eating habits, consistently getting a good night's sleep, exercising regularly, and pursuing medical treatment to address long-term health issues.

If you are constantly depressed, you may want to seek a doctor's advice. But while you are at it, why not see a psychotherapist and get to the bottom of your depression? An even better idea might be to see a therapist who practices positive psychology. From what we've read, it's a more effective way of building a better life than spending months dredging up horrid memories of your past and trying to come to grips with them. To learn about this relatively new field of psychology, check out *The Happiness Advantage* by Shawn Achor. It's one of Dan's favorite books on the subject.

Also psychologists claim that talking with close friends and loved ones about the trials and tribulations of your life can help you feel better. You may want to even seek a nutritionist's advice to improve your diet and how you feel. Aerobic exercise for at least 20 minutes three times a week can also reduce stress. We've both found this to be extremely helpful over the years. We'd also recommend you read the book *Brain Food* by Dr. Lisa Mosconi. It's a guide to achieving mental health by providing your brain the nutrients it needs to thrive.

If you think you have something medically wrong with you like a sluggish set of adrenal glands or a tired thyroid, seek medical help. Get a diagnosis from a competent physician or, perhaps even better, a naturopathic doctor who practices holistic medicine. If you go the MD route, try to find a doctor who practices holistic medicine or integrated medicine – that is, one who looks for multiple causes and treats the root causes of what ails patients, not just the symptoms like most MDs.

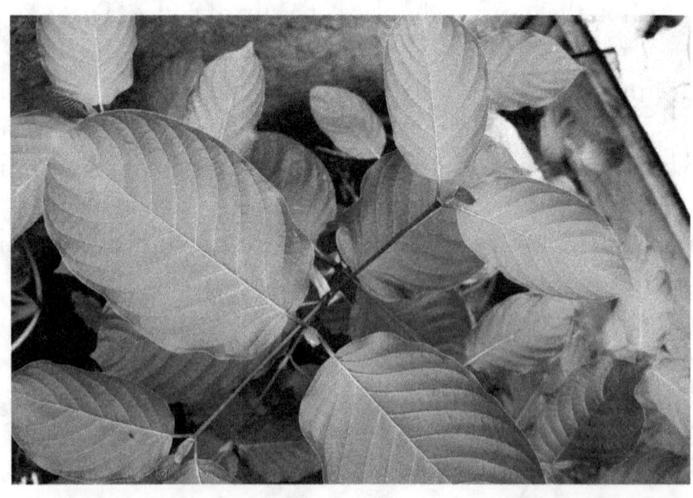

A FEW WORDS OF
CAUTION

We're not medical experts but know that it is sound advice when Kratom authors advise people not to ever mix WVK with any other stimulants like amphetamines. Caffeine, some say, may be an exception. Even then, it's always a good idea to not mix chemical substances that have the same effect. Start slowly, taking two to three grams of Kratom at first to assess the effect. If you're a tiny person, you may want to take even less. If you weigh more, you may want to try a slightly larger dose, but always err on the cautious side.

To carefully study your body's reaction to Kratom, try taking it at the same time of day and under the same conditions, for example, in the morning on an empty or a full stomach. Be consistent. That is, take it the same time and same way each time (e.g., by capsule on an empty stomach) initially as you experiment with effects it has on your body. Adjust accordingly.

Remember also, that it takes time for Kratom's active ingredients to get into your bloodstream. Don't expect immediate effects. How you take Kratom (capsule vs. powder) and whether or not you are taking it on an empty stomach will greatly affect its absorption into your bloodstream. Even the time of day and your body weight may affect the amount of time it takes to feel an effect.

What about green-vein Kratom?

The **effects of green-veined Kratom (GVK), lie somewhere in the middle of RVK and WVK.** That is to say, it provides benefits of both. For example, GVK **improves mood, boosts energy levels, and soothes pain** like RVK. You may very likely feel **more at ease, peaceful, and calm**, but you will find yourself **being motivated and able to work harder, an effect of WVK.** You may find yourself being **more talkative, more cheerful, friendlier, and noticeably more extroverted.** Dan really noticed this effect. It's kind of cool.

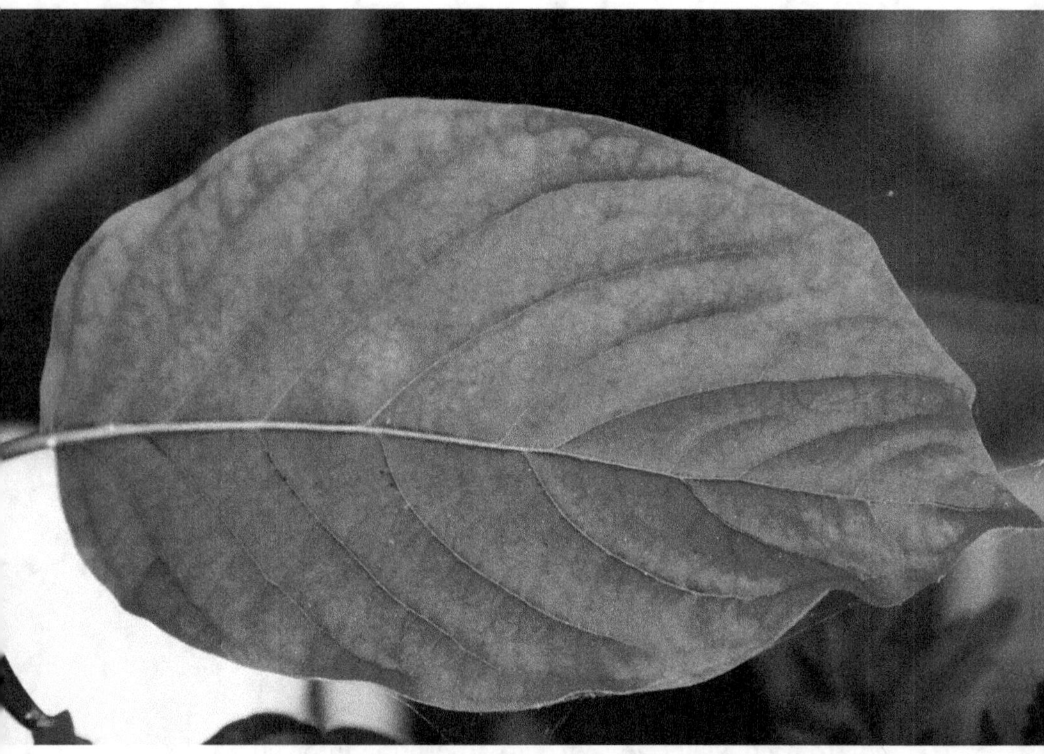

Part of the joyful feeling you get stems from the fact that you'll be very likely to care a whole lot less about what others think of you. In other words, you may be more comfortable in your own skin, which in and of itself is a great feeling.

GVK is often used when individuals are going to parties or will be involved in other social settings like conferences that ordinarily make them uncomfortable. **GVK makes people feel braver, less timid, friendlier, more cheerful, and more talkative.**

Is there a yellow-veined Kratom?

As you search for product, you will also encounter vendors who sell yellow Kratom. Some even label their product "yellow-veined Kratom." What's up with this?

Yellow-veined Kratom (YVK) is a relative newcomer to the Kratom family that some authors think may be slowly conquering the market. It's one of our favorites. It has an effect between red and white.

First things first: there is no such thing as a yellow-veined Kratom leaf. You won't find yellow-veined leaves growing on plants.

How is Yellow Kratom made?

There's quite a lot of debate as to how yellow Kratom (YK) is made. Rather than confuse you with the different thoughts, let's go with the majority opinion, the most common explanation we've encountered.

Most authors think YK is produced by altering the drying process of all three types of leaves: red, green, and white. For example, if RVK leaves are dried longer when making RVK, the veins turn yellow. Green- or white-veined leaves dried outdoors (rather than inside) in the Sun also turn yellow. In addition, dried leaves may also be fermented to produce YK.

These treatments do not just change the color of the leaves' veins, they alter the mixture of alkaloids in the final product.

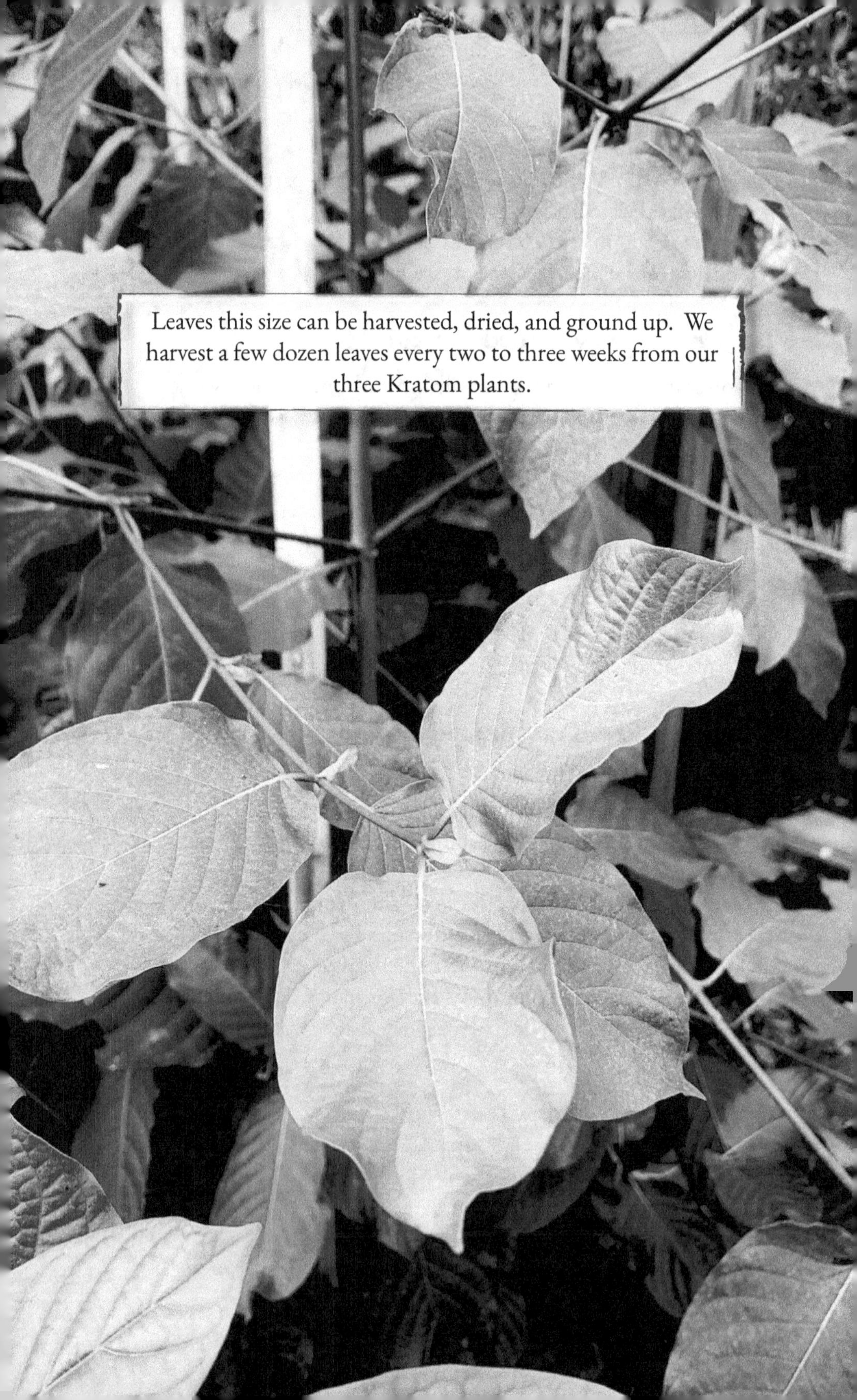

Leaves this size can be harvested, dried, and ground up. We
harvest a few dozen leaves every two to three weeks from our
three Kratom plants.

05

PROCEED WITH CAUTION: ASSESING YOUR REACTIONS TO KRATOM

What factors should you take into account when assessing your reaction to Kratom?

The benefits and side effects one reaps and experiences, respectively, from all types of medicines, including herbal supplements like Kratom, depends on a great many factors.

What's the most important determinant of beneficial effects and unwanted side effects?

One of the most important factors that determines how a person responds to -- both positively and negatively -- to Kratom is the dose – that is, how much one takes at any one time.

Low doses of Kratom (3 to 5 grams) may result in one effect, for example, they may calm you down. Higher doses (approximately 6 to 10 grams) of the same type of Kratom, however, may prove to be a somnolent, lulling you into sleep. Even higher doses may bring about an entirely different effect, so be careful.

What other factors affect your body's response to Kratom?

The effect one experiences also depends on two additional factors, not often discussed in Kratom books: your age and body weight. Younger people may respond differently than older people. Lighter individuals may respond to the same dose differently than those who are carrying more weight.

Another factor that could influence your reaction is your mental and physical state. If you are tired, for example, you might respond differently than if you are feeling excited or, perhaps, hyped up on coffee.

Yet another factor is the time of day. You may respond to a medicinal herb like Kratom different in the morning than you would in the afternoon or evening. That's partly due to the fact that energy levels often vary during the day. It's also partly due to the fact that physiology varies throughout the day thanks in large part to naturally occurring daily hormonal cycles.

Your health status may also affect your response. Are you feeling well or feeling under the weather?

Yet another factor is your genetics. Remember, we are not all genetically identical. Our genes affect how our bodies react to all kinds of things from heat and humidity to prescription medicines. Kratom could also be influenced by one's genetic makeup. Differences in genetics could result in differences in liver function that in turn affect how quickly a medicinal herb's active ingredients are catabolized (broken down) and eliminated via the excretory system.

Last but not least in the list of possible influencers is sex. Men and women are quite different physiological creatures. The many differences in our metabolism and hormonal production could also influence how we react to Kratom.

That's a lot to keep in mind when taking a medicine of any kind. But it's important to be mindful of the fact that you may react entirely differently to Kratom than someone else, even another family member. If so, you have a list of possible reasons.

Are any factors more important than others?

We think, dose, body weight, time of day, and emotional and physical state are the most important factors to consider when taking any medicine, Kratom included.

How long does it take to feel the effects of Kratom?

The effects you feel when taking Kratom may commence in as few as 10 to 20 minutes – perhaps even within 5 minutes -- or as long as 30 to 40 minutes, according to various sources we've read and our own personal experience. We've found that the effects usually come on very subtly. That is, they kind of sneak up on you in a pleasant way.

Why does the onset of beneficial affects vary?

The onset of beneficial effects depends on several factors. The most important factor is the form in which you ingest Kratom.

If you prepare Kratom tea and drink it down fairly quickly, for instance, you will very likely feel the effects more rapidly – easily with 5 to 10 minutes. Dan's noticed an effect within minutes after drinking Kratom tea made from dried, crushed leaves or powder.

Liquid carriers like tea result in a rapid response because the active ingredients are quickly absorbed into the bloodstream through the small intestine. They are then rapidly transported throughout your body via the cardiovascular system.

If you ingest Kratom as a powder or paste – as many people do -- and then wash it down with water or some other liquid, like orange juice or chocolate milk, you will very likely feel the effects rather quickly as well -- and for the same reason.

If you ingest Kratom in capsule form, you may feel the benefits a little more slowly. That's because it takes a little bit of time for the capsule to break down, and the active ingredients to be transported to the first segment of the small intestine where it is absorbed into the bloodstream.

Does response time have anything to do with the amount of food in your stomach?

Another key factor in determining the time in which effects begin is how much food is in your stomach. Most people are familiar with this phenomenon because alcohol's effects vary with stomach contents. Kratom is no different. How quickly the active ingredients of Kratom are absorbed into the bloodstream depends on how much food is in the stomach and small intestine. If you are taking Kratom in any form on an empty stomach, you'll could feel the effects more quickly than if your stomach's full.

What about your mental or physiological status?

Your mental status can also affect the onset of effects. If you are super excited or happy and take a Kratom product that increases energy levels, you may feel the effects more rapidly than if you are down in the dumps or worn out from a long, tiring day at work.

Your physiological status can play a role. If you just woke up from a restful sleep, your response may be much faster than if you woke up groggy after a rotten night's sleep. Bear in mind that most of us suffer from fatigue late in the afternoon. Our biorhythms are down. We also often feel groggy after a meal like lunch. That feeling is referred to as the post prandial (after-eating) slump. During such times response rates may be slower.

Caffeine ingestion may also affect the onset of Kratoms effects. If you are hyped up on caffeine or cruising along on a high level of adrenalin from stress and ingest a red-veined Kratom product to calm yourself down, it may take a little longer to feel Kratom's calming effects than if you are feeling more tranquil. (It also might take a higher dose of Kratom.)

Keep these factors in mind when gauging your reaction time. That is, be mindful of your state of mind and body. Don't take more Kratom if the desired effect doesn't manifest itself right away. Be patient.

How long do the effects last?

Kratom's a rather long-lasting botanical medicine. Most people say they enjoy the benefits for around four or five hours. Some people claim up to six hours.

Are there any side effects to Kratom?

Just like any other chemical substance you ingest or inhale, Kratom may have undesirable side effects. The side effects one feels vary with dose and the type of Kratom you are taking. As noted earlier, Dan and Linda both notice slightly reduced mental acuity and sluggish memory after taking red-veined Kratom capsules, but not with white-veined Kratom products.

The list of possible side effects we've found in our readings from different Kratom may include:

- Nausea
- Itching
- Sweating
- Dry mouth
- Constipation
- Diarrhea
- Increased urination
- Loss of appetite

What are the signs that someone has taken too much — that is, overdosed on Kratom?

All medications – even Tylenol and Ibuprofen when taken in excess – can result in adverse side effects – sometimes horrible side effects. Kratom's no exception. From the sources we've consulted, overdosing may result in one or more of the following symptoms:

- Muscle pain
- Chills
- Dry mouth
- Nausea and vomiting
- Dizziness
- Drowsiness
- Heightened sensitivity to UV radiation

Are there any side effects from the long-term use of high doses?

Studies of frequent Kratom users in Thailand and Malaysia suggest some adverse long-term side effects occur in individuals taking high doses of Kratom for prolonged periods.

They may include:

- Weight loss
- Insomnia (defined as difficulty falling asleep or staying asleep)
- Hyperpigmentation (dark spots) on the skin, especially on the cheeks
- Fatigue
- Constipation
- Nausea

- Loss of appetite
- Frequent urination
- Dry mouth
- Tremors or shaking
- Seizures
- Psychosis (seeing or hearing things that others do not see or hear)

High doses of Kratom are not recommended. Prolonged high-dose treatments are even less advisable. If you ignore this advice and are experiencing any of these side effects, you should contact your healthcare provider at once or head to an urgent care center or an emergency room. Be honest and upfront. Let the doctors know right away.

Should children or pregnant women take Kratom.

The American Kratom Association, an industry organization dedicated to the safe production and use of Kratom, says no. Absolutely not. There's not enough known about the risks of exposing pregnant women and their embryos or fetuses to Kratom. The same goes with children under the age of 18.

Will Kratom react with other prescription medications or illicit drugs?

In an online article in Everyday Health, Lindsey Konkel writes: "In February 2018, the FDA released the details of 44 deaths that had been associated with Kratom use. In all but one case, fatality reports indicated that users had mixed Kratom with other prescription or illegal drugs, including benzodiazepines (ben-zoe-die-az-ah-peens) and Tramadol."

Benzodiazepines is a class of drugs that includes some of the most commonly prescribed medications in the United States. Some benzodiazepines are prescribed as **muscle relaxants**. Other formulations are prescribed to help patients **relieve anxiety and insomnia.** Still other benzodiazepines are used to **help alcoholics lessen withdrawal symptoms.** Others are given to patients as an anesthetic before certain procedures or surgeries. Tramadol is an opioid taken for moderate to severe pain.

Here's a list of benzodiazepine drugs:

- Alprazolam (Xanax)
- Clonazepam (Klonopin)
- Clorazepate (Tranxene)
- Diazepam (Valium)
- Estazolam (Prosom)
- Flurazepam (Dalmane)
- Lorazepam (Ativan)
- Midazolam (Versed)
- Oxazepam (Serax)
- Temazepam (Restoril)
- Triazolam (Halcion)
- Quazepam (Doral)

Konkel goes on to say, "It's not clear yet exactly which drugs may be safe to use while taking Kratom or which combinations could cause health problems. More research is needed to understand how Kratom interacts with over-the-counter and prescription medication and other drugs..."

Because so little is known about drug interactions, many sources recommend that Kratom users not take it with any other prescription medications or any other illegal drug.

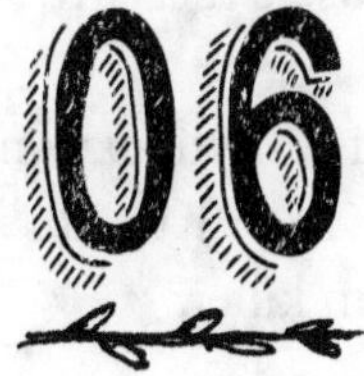

HOW DO KRATOMS PHYTOCHEMICALS WORK?

What are Kratom's active ingredients and what do they do?

As noted earlier, the Kratom leaf is nature's drugstore -- chock full of potentially beneficial ingredients.

Mitragynine (MG) is the most prevalent alkaloid, comprising about 66% of the alkaloids found in Kratom. Research suggests that mitragynine is primarily responsible for blocking pain as well as the stimulatory effects of Kratom.

Next in line is an alkaloid called **paynanthine** (pay-nan-theen). It comprises about 9% of all the alkaloids. (Scientists are not sure what it does.)

Third in line, with respect to abundance, is a chemical called

speciogynine (spee-see-oh-guy-neen). It comprises about 7% of the alkaloid population. It's a muscle relaxant.

Another important alkaloid is **7-hydroxy mitragynine** (7-HM). The compound comprises about 2% of Kratom's total alkaloid production and, like mitragynine, is a pain killer.

Here's what's important about 7-HM: Even though it is found in lesser quantities, 7-HM is much more potent than MG. In fact, 7-HM is considered *the* most potent analgesic (pain killer) of the alkaloid's found in Kratom.

Are the alkaloids the only beneficial phytochemicals in Kratom?

Kratom contains a lot of other phytochemicals besides alkaloids that could very likely play key roles in promoting better health. These beneficial phytochemicals are found in a number of other plants.

The best example is **epicatechin** (ep-a-cat-eh-chin). Epicatechin is no stranger to the plant world. It's one of the beneficial phytochemicals found in dark chocolate, green tea, and cranberries.

Epicatechin offers many health benefits. It is, for example, a **strong antioxidant** that helps protect us again cancer. As an antioxidant, it also helps prevent atherosclerosis (hardening of the arteries) that often lead to heart attacks and strokes. Research suggests that epicatechin **may also impair the growth of potentially pathogenic bacteria.** It can be used to treat urinary tract infections (that's why natural medicine savvy individuals tell us to drink cranberry juice when you've got a UTI).

How does Kratom relieve pain?

According to research performed by the US Food and Drug Administration (FDA), Kratom relieves pain because some of its alkaloids, notably MG and 7-HMG, bind to naturally occurring opioid receptors in the body. In doing so, they block pain. These alkaloids are naturally occurring opioids. **(Some readers may object to this designation, opioids are, by definition, chemical substances that bind to opioid receptors.)** Its opioid components have prompted the FDA to consider actions to ban Kratom -- no doubt at the urging of Big Pharma (All this occurs, while legal prescription opioids kill tens of thousands of Americans each year). The next question is:

Because Kratom contains opioids is it dangerous?

When we first heard that Kratom contains opioids, we were surprised and wary. Let's face it, opioids have been front page news for quite a while. Just the word opioid evokes fear, and for good reason. In 2019, for instance, there were 50,042 reported deaths in the United States caused by opioid overdose.

Concerned, we began to research this issue. One of the first things we learned was that the body produces its own opioids. That's why we have opioid receptors in the first place. In fact, the body has three different types of opioid receptors called Mu, Delta, and Kappa receptors. Naturally produced opioids bind to these receptors, blocking pain and creating a feeling of well-being.

The best known of the body's natural opioids is a group known as endorphins. Endorphins are synthesized and released by the brain and the pituitary gland when we experience pain. They then circulate throughout the bloodstream and bind to opioid receptors in nerve cells throughout the body, suppressing pain. You can think of them as nature's way of suppressing pain signals.

Endorphins are also released during exercise, orgasm, and when we eat delicious food, promoting a general sense of euphoria. The runner's high you may have heard about is the result of endorphins released during a long run in the park.

Endorphins are not the only natural pain killers, however. The body also produces two lesser known opioids, known as enkephalins and dynorphins.

So, the first thing to think about is this: If the human body produces it's own opioids, it's clear that not all opioids are bad. From what we've read, the opioids found in Kratom are not as dangerous as heroin, morphine, and other opioids commonly overused and misused today. One research study on mice showed that unlike heroin and other opioids, Kratom may not suppress respiration as much as drugs like morphine. Respiratory depression is the number one killer of individuals who overdose on medical and illicit opioids. We'll explore these and other topics in Chapter 9, which delves into the safety of Kratom.

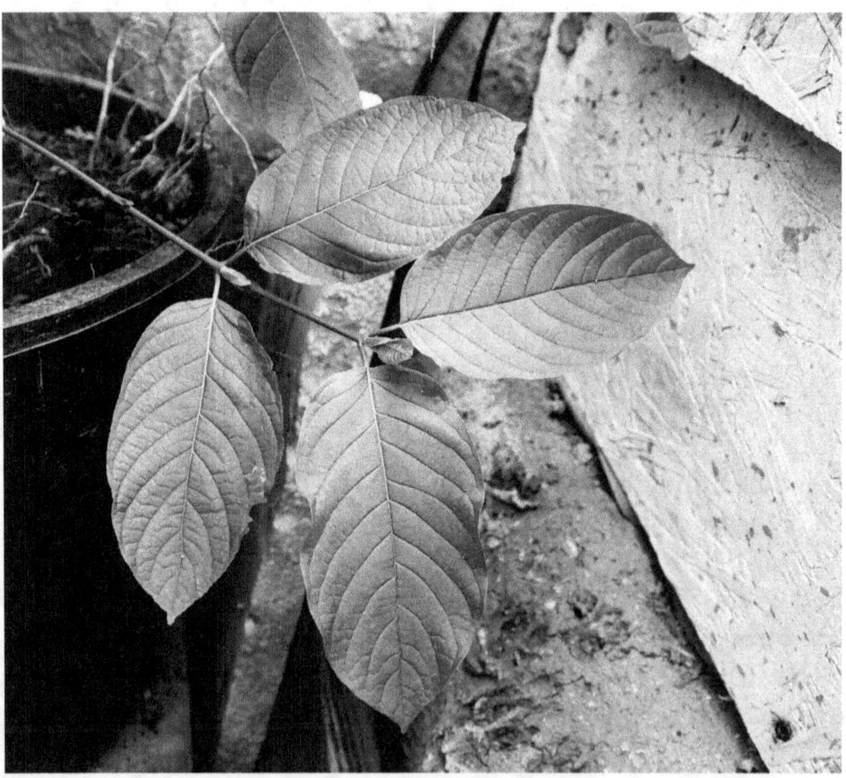

07

PROCEED CAREFULLY: PURCHASING KRATOM

Where can I purchase Kratom?

Kratom is becoming increasingly available in the United States and other nations. In the US, you can purchase it at convenience stores and other retail outlets, for example, those that sell CBD products. Be careful, though. Not all producers are ethical. The widest selection of reliable products like capsules and power are available on the Internet. Look for companies that have been around for a while and have good reviews.

What forms does it come in?

Kratom comes in many forms, including (1) partially ground leaves, (2) finely ground powder, (3) capsules filled with powder, and (4) pills made from powder or a concentrated leaf extract. Let's take a look at each one.

Kratom leaves can be partially ground much like tea leaves. They can be used to make Kratom tea, a topic we discuss in detail in Chapter 8. Partially ground leaves can also be further ground, creating a finely ground powder. Powders, in turn, can be ingested in one of several ways, for example, they can placed in water or some other liquid, stirred then swallowed. They can also be boiled to create a hot tea or placed in capsules (more on all of this in Chapter 8).

By far the most popular forms of Kratom are powder and capsules. You'll pay a little more for capsules, but they're a lot more convenient.

How do you find a reputable source of Kratom?

There are numerous reliable sources of Kratom on the Internet. Your challenge is to find one.

We discovered the brand we use through a person we trusted. He recommended a supplier from which a number of his acquaintances were purchasing Kratom. (They were taking Kratom to relieve chronic pain from arthritis.) We purchased some sample packs of Kratom powder – white, red, and green powder – from that company.

As a side note: The company from which we purchased Kratom was EZ Kratom. We're not endorsing the company and its products, just stating that we've found the company and their Kratom powder to be quite good.

If you've been watching the nightly news lately, you've noticed that a small number of unscrupulous players is causing serious problems in the CBD market. Some disreputable sources are peddling products that fall short of company promises – their products contain less CBD than advertised or none at all. Still others are selling CBD oils that have way more THC than they're supposed to. In worst cases, some disreputable companies have laced their products with potentially poisonous chemicals.

Similar crooked practices exist in the Kratom business. Experience has shown that some shysters who are out to make a quick buck lace their products with potentially harmful chemicals. There's been at least one incidence of Kratom containing harmful bacteria. Although, we haven't heard of any cases in which "fake" Kratom powder was sold to customers, it is bound to happen.

How do you pay for your purchases?

Kratom is legal in most cities, countries, and states. Despite its legal status, you can't purchase Kratom with a credit or debit card. Reputable suppliers won't offer that option. Why?

Basically, it boils down to this. Kratom is considered a high-risk product by the US banking industry. Consequently, US banks forbid vendors from making sales of Kratom via plastic.

Although some international banks allow the sale of Kratom on their end, some US banks won't allow international payments for Kratom to clear or will charge an additional fee.

When shopping for Kratom, beware: New online Kratom vendors sellers may allow payments through PayPal, Square, Stripe, Venmo, and Amazon Payments. Unfortunately, these processors also view Kratom as a "high-risk product." Selling Kratom violates their terms and conditions. When Kratom sales are detected, PayPal and others can freeze a vendor's account for up to six months. If you have just placed an order, these companies will very likely hold the money you deposited in the vendor's account when making the purchase. You will most likely not receive the product you ordered in the near term – perhaps forever. Moreover, there's a chance that you will not receive a refund -- even though the vendor was at fault. So, what's a person to do?

Needless to say, payment options are limited. One option is COD (cash on delivery). When the product arrives, you pay the Post Office. They, in turn, give the money to the seller.

Another is a direct transfer from your checking account to the vendors. Banks do this all the time – for example, they allow customers to pay bills online automatically each month. The money is withdrawn directly from your checking account.

Direct transfer, however, is be a bit scary and potentially quite risky. For Kratom purchases, you'll need to provide the Kratom dealer with banking information so they can access your checking account to withdraw your payment.

To reduce risk when we started buying Kratom, we used a checking account that typically had very little money in it. That way, if the company scammed us, we wouldn't be hurt too badly. Fortunately, the company from which we purchased Kratom (EZ Kratom) was true to their word. After we established an account with them and provided the information they needed for a direct transfer, they withdrew the amount we owed them. Nothing more, nothing less. They shipped the product the same day the payment cleared. (Bear in mind, it will take a few days to set up the transfer.)

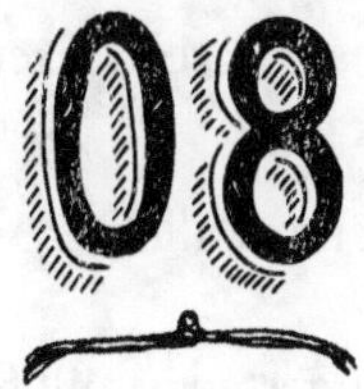

METHODS OF INGESTION

Is there anything you should know before you decide on a method of ingestion?

Absolutely. Like many herbal meds, Kratom isn't the best-tasting stuff in the Universe. It may be especially distasteful to individuals who are sensitive to bitter flavors. To Dan, Kratom powder and leaves taste awful. If you're like him, capsules may be the best option.

Linda and others we've talked to don't mind the taste. Linda wouldn't drink it for pleasure, but it's not that bad as an herbal medicine. Remarkably, some people like the taste of Kratom. To them, it is like Matcha tea.

You'll have to try it to see.

Fortunately, there are ways to make Kratom more palatable. Kratom teas made from leaves or powders, for instance, can be sweetened with honey or some other sweetener. Mixing Kratom powder into smoothies or shakes or with ice cream can also hide the taste. (more on this shortly.)

How do people ingest Kratom?

There are lots of ways to ingest Kratom. Here's a fairly comprehensive list:

- Kratom capsules can be swallowed with a liquid like water or orange juice.
- Kratom can also be ingested in pill form, though, there aren't many vendors who sell pills.
- Kratom powder can be placed in the mouth, then washed down with a liquid such as orange juice or chocolate milk – this is the "toss and wash method."

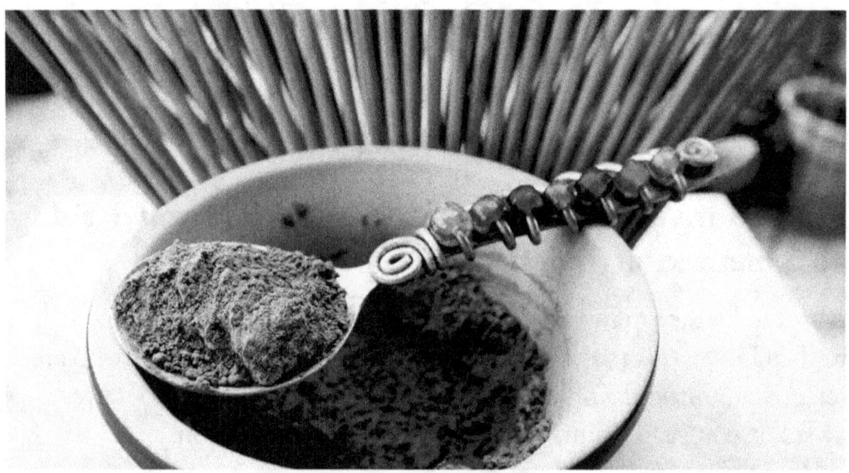

- Kratom powder can be placed in the mouth, sloshed around a bit with a teaspoon of water or juice, then washed down with a liquid such as orange juice or chocolate milk. A second or third dose may be required, depending on the dose. An additional swallow or two may help rid your mouth of any unswallowed powder. We call this the "toss, slosh and wash method."
- Kratom powder can be mixed with water and made into a paste, placed in the mouth, then washed down with a liquid.
- Kratom powder can be mixed with drinks like chocolate milk or chocolate almond milk or foods like ice cream,

yogurt, or fruit smoothies, then consumed.
- Kratom leaves can be used to make tea, then sweetened to taste, if necessary (To Linda sweetening heightens the taste, making it less palatable. To Dan sweetening the tea makes Kratom quite palatable.)
- Kratom powder can be used to make tea, which can be sweetened
- Highly concentrated Kratom extract pills can be swallowed.
- Kratom leaves can be smoked.

What is the most palatable way to take Kratom?

By far, the most palatable way to ingest Kratom if you are sensitive to the taste of its alkaloids is taking it in capsule form. You can take capsules with any drink, although alcoholic beverages aren't recommended.

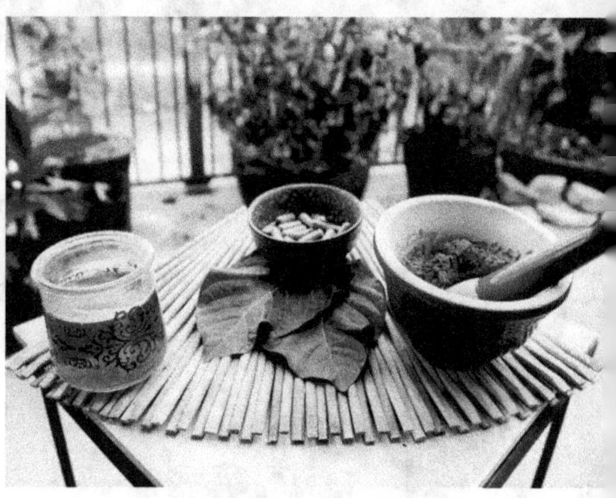

Tell me more about capsules

Kratom powder is the most widely sold product online. However, you can purchase capsules from some suppliers, although there are fewer online vendors who sell capsules than powders.

Although capsuled Kratom is a bit more expensive, it is by far the easiest way to painlessly avail yourself to the beneficial effects of this herbal medicine.

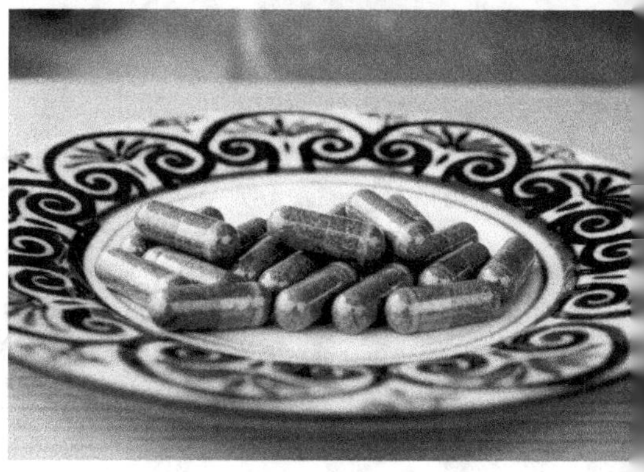

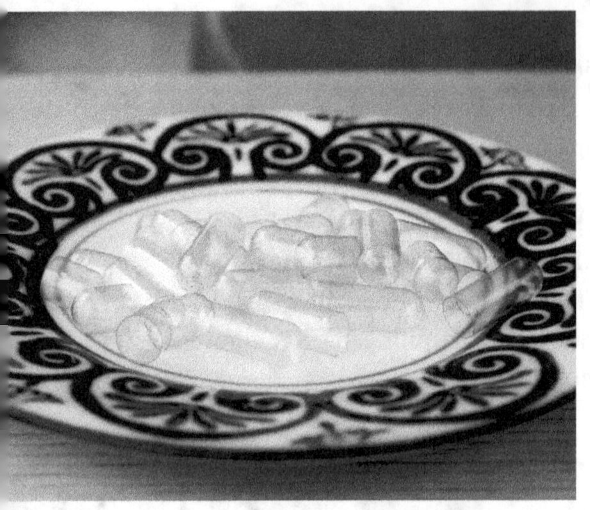

Another option is to buy Kratom powder, and then fill capsules yourself, preferably with a capsule machine like the one shown below. Capsule machines typically make up to 100 capsules at a time. They're relatively inexpensive too, costing between $15 and $35.

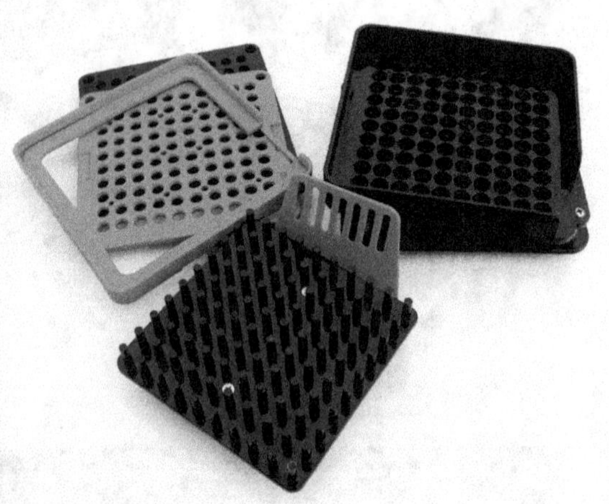

Making your own capsules is a bit time consuming and messy. Be sure to wear gloves and a face mask if you're making your own capsules. Also place some clean white paper on the surface you are working on to catch and recover powder that invariably spills out of the capsule machine.

Capsules come in a variety of different sizes. Most capsules on the market are size 000 or 00.

- 000 size contains about 1.0 gram of Kratom powder
- 00 size capsules contain about 0.75 grams powder
- 0 size capsules contain 0.5 grams of Kratom powder
- 1 size capsules contain about 0.4 grams of Kratom powder
- 2 size capsules contain about 0.3 grams of Kratom powder

We use size 00, the most widely available capsule.

Should I buy preseparated capsules or unseparated capsules?

As you search the Internet for capsules, you'll find there are two major types. Some manufacturers sell capsules that are "pre-separated," that is, they are not assembled. You'll receive two packages of capsule halves, one bag with the large end of the capsule and the other with the smaller segment. Many companies sell unseparated capsules, that is, empty assembled capsules. Unseparated capsules are a pain in the neck, as they have to be manually separated before they can be used. This can be time consuming. **So, shop carefully. We've found that a vast majority of suppliers sell unseparated capsules.**

So, be sure to check whether capsules are separated or unseparated. It's odd, but many manufacturers don't tell you up front whether their capsules are pre-separated. You usually can find this information in the Q and A section of their page on vendors like Amazon.

Most capsules are made from gelatin, an animal byproduct; are there any options for vegans or vegetarians?

Capsules are made from either plant or animal matter.

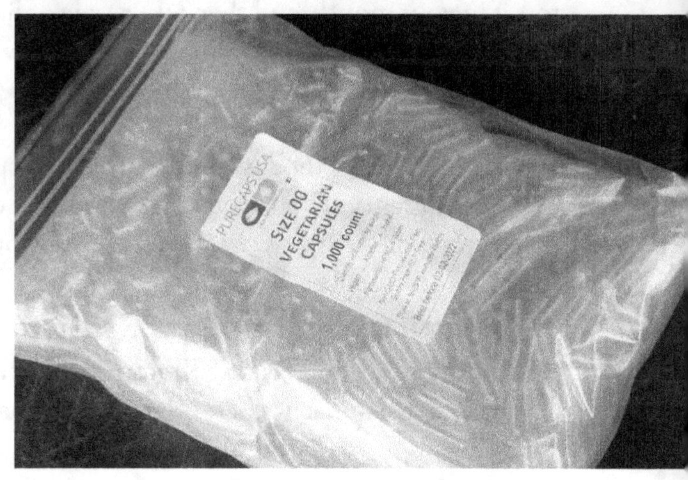

PURECAPS USA, for instance, sells capsules that are made from plant material. As a result, they're vegan, kosher, and Halal. They're also nonGMA, preservative-free, and gluten-free, in case you are interested.

We purchase this brand.

Most capsules are made from animal matter, notably, gelatin. Gelatin is a colorless, flavorless material made from collagen; a type of protein found in animals' connective tissue.

Is Kratom powder recommended?

Some authors argue that Kratom powder is the best product on the market. That's primarily because it is readily available and cheaper than capsules. Another advantage of powder is that there are a lot more varieties of Kratom powder on the market than capsules, creating wider choice. (Let's be frank, though, early on, you'll very likely want to stick to a few choices. You can get confused very quickly, so initially it's probably best to purchase one type of red, one type of white, and one type of green.)

How is Kratom powder ingested?

The simplest way to ingest Kratom powder is to take a single teaspoon, toss it in your mouth, and then take a swig of liquid, slosh it around, and then swallow. You may want to wash it down with water, chocolate milk, or orange juice.

When using this method, remember that a teaspoon of Kratom weighs about four grams. If you are taking a moderate dose of Kratom, say 8 grams, you will need to repeat the process. I wouldn't place all 8 grams in my mouth at once.

> A word of warning: Taking Kratom via the toss and wash method, may invite stomach aches. If it does, you may want to invest in a capsule-making machine.

Is there an easier way to take Kratom powder?

If the idea of ingesting a dry powder is not appealing, you can convert Kratom powder into a paste and swallow that. To make a paste, place the desired amount of Kratom, say one or two teaspoons, in a coffee cup. Add a little hot water and mix it to create a paste.

When the paste is done, place one-half to one teaspoon of Kratom in your mouth and then chase it with a drink of water or some other liquid. (Again, you may want to slosh it around a wee bit in your mouth before swallowing.) When starting out, you may want to swallow a half teaspoon at a time.

What about Kratom slurries?

Another option for taking Kratom is to create a slurry. A slurry is a liquid with Kratom powder suspended in it.

Here's how you make it: Mix the amount of Kratom you want to take in water, stir it very well, and when it is well suspended, take a drink. Add more water and stir it once again, then swallow the remaining powder.

Another option is to place Kratom powder in a small container with a lid. Shake vigorously, then drink it down – all at once or in a couple portions. When the cup, glass, or container is empty, add some more water to suspend the clumps sticking to the side of the container. Shake or stir the powder into solution, then chug it down.

Please note that some people chase slurries with orange juice or some other sweet-flavored drink to get the awful taste out of their mouths.

How hard is it to mix Kratom powder with liquids?

Kratom powder can be mixed with water and a variety of water-based beverages, such as cow's milk, orange juice, and soy drink. Unfortunately, Kratom is not very water soluble. When mixed with cold water or milk, for example, it tends to form clumps. To break them up, you will have to stir vigorously. This helps to keep the powder suspended in solution. Even so, when you've finished your Kratom drink, you will find small gobs of the green sticky paste clinging to the wall and bottom of your glass or mug. To remove it, you'll need to add more liquid, and vigorously stir or shake the mixture again to dislodge them. Even after a second mix, you may find some clingons.

When mixed with hot water, we've found that powder goes into solution better -- that is some of the active ingredients dissolve in hot water, creating a green-colored liquid. In addition, warm liquids tend to create a better suspension of insoluble particles. Even so, a thin layer of water-insoluble powder will precipitate on the bottom of your cup. You can decant the liquid and discard the powder or drink it all down to get the full benefits of the Kratom. As noted earlier, you may need to add sweetener to the mix to make it more palatable.

I'm told Kratom mixes well with chocolate milk, is that true?

As just noted, Kratom's not very water soluble. However, it does blend more easily with chocolate milk. The chocolate flavoring (and sugar) mask the foul taste of Kratom, and the creamy texture of chocolate milk helps suspend the Kratom particles in solution. Although some Kratom will settle out of solution, it won't do so as quickly as it does when mixed in water or most other liquids.

To try this method, add your Kratom to a cup of chocolate milk. Stir well, then add more chocolate milk. Stir again. If it's not fully suspended, add a little more chocolate and stir again. You could even pour the mix into a blender to see if that helps.

Can you mix Kratom with food?

Absolutely.

Kratom can be blended into ice cream, pudding, applesauce, or yogurt...pretty much any creamy food. You can add it to a smoothie, or a protein shake. Foods such as these can be a great vehicle for getting this stuff down your gullet. Sweeteners in these foods do a good job of masking the flavor of Kratom.

We've tried Kratom with a couple different types of ice cream. In our "experiments" with chocolate and orange swirl ice cream, we have found that ice cream does a pretty good job of negating the taste of the Kratom powder -- and vice versa. If you didn't catch that sneaky vice versa, let us say it another way. Kratom does a great job of negating the flavor of a delicious bowl of ice cream. Ice cream isn't going to taste awful, but it isn't going to taste at all like it should. (Linda considers this method a pretty good way to ruin a delicious bowl of ice cream.)

How do you make a Kratom smoothie or shake?

The easiest way to make a smoothie is to fill a blender with the fruits and vegetables you like, then add a little fruit juice, milk, soy beverage, or other liquid. Add ice, too, if desired. Next add the amount of powder you deem appropriate, place the cover on the blender and turn it on. Let it run until the concoction you've created can be justly called a smoothie.

Needless to say, you can try lots of different fruits such as apples, bananas, peaches, and berries. Lots of different vegetables can be added as well, including chopped spinach or kale.

Protein shakes are another great vehicle for imbibing Kratom. Follow your favorite recipes, but add Kratom.

Kratom oatmeal anyone?

Sure, why not?

Some people mix Kratom powder with regular or instant oatmeal. Cook according to instructions and sweeten to taste. Add whatever you like to make the oatmeal "your way" – for example, soy beverage, milk, butter, brown sugar, nuts or berries.

How is Kratom powder used to make hot tea?

As noted earlier, Kratom powder and partially ground leaves can be used to make teas. Fortunately, there are a lot of options when it comes to preparing hot Kratom teas. Here's the simplest method when using powder: First, add Kratom powder to boiling hot water – one teaspoon per cup gives you 4 grams. Let it steep for 10 to 15 minutes. Stir occasionally.

During this process many of the soluble beneficial phytochemicals will dissolve into solution. The insoluble materials will settle on the bottom.

Next, add the desired amount of sweetener – for example, honey or erythritol, a healthy sweetener -- to make the drink palatable, then stir it in, and drink it hot – bottom sludge (undissolved powder on the bottom) and all.

Can you mix Kratom powder with commercially available forms of tea?

Absolutely.

Take the recipe I just gave you for Kratom tea but immerse a bag of your favorite tea in the solution while your Kratom tea is steeping. You can try any tea, including green tea, chamomile, peppermint – whatever suits your fancy. Sweeten it however you want, too.

What about cold tea?

If you want to make a straight-Kratom iced tea, mix the Kratom powder in hot water – as many cups as you want to make. (Be sure to keep track of the amount of Kratom you add per cup.). Stir it, then let it steep for 10 to 15 minutes.

When the mix has cooled, pour the liquid into another container like a pitcher. You can leave the undissolved powder on the bottom of the first container, then wash it down the drain or pour it into a compost pile. Or you can stir it up and add it to the pitcher.

If needed, sweeten your tea at this time or wait until you're ready to drink it.

Next, place the pitcher in the fridge and consume it to your heart's delight. **Be careful, though. If you've added three teaspoons of Kratom powder per cup of hot water, don't drink two cups at a time.** You'll be ingesting 12 grams at one sitting. Needless to say, you should keep Kratom tea out of reach of children, teens, and anyone else you want.

How do you make Kratom tea from dried leaves?

As noted earlier, dried Kratom leaves can also be used to make tea. Tea leaves can be immersed directly in water or in a tea ball infuser, then allowed to steep. This is a quick method of ingesting Kratom that's ideal for people growing their own Kratom.

If you want to experiment, you can also add other types of teas like peppermint or orange spice to the mix to create a unique blend that tickles your fancy. Sweeten to taste.

I've heard about Kratom extract. What is it?

Kratom extract is a concentrated Kratom product. It's made by mixing powder or crushed leaves in liquid, boiling the mix, then decanting (pouring off) the liquid. The supernatant (liquid without leaves or powder) is then boiled down to form a highly concentrated paste. The paste can then be dried and converted into a powder. The highly concentrated powder can then be encapsulated or used to make pills.

Watch out! Concentrates such as this can be quite strong. **Extracts you purchase online, for instance, may contain ten or fifteen times**

the amount of active ingredients found in an equal volume of powder. One gram of 10x extract contains the same amount of active ingredients as 10 grams of powder. That's a substantial dose. One gram of 15x extract contains the same quantity of active ingredients as 15 grams of powder. That's a very high dose.

So, it's worth reiterating: if you use Kratom extract of any kind, homemade or purchased from the Internet, be very careful. Not only is it powerful, but commercially available concentrates could be laced with potentially harmful substances when purchased from unscrupulous vendors.

Can Kratom be smoked?

Kratom leaves can be dried, then partially crushed and mixed with another form of dried leaf, like tobacco, then rolled and smoked.

There's one problem with this technique, however. You'll never know how much Kratom is in a leaf, so dosing becomes problematic.

Moreover, smoking is a quick way to ruin your lungs. Sulfur compounds in smoke from cigarettes, marijuana, and Kratom leaf are converted to sulfur dioxide gas during combustion. When inhaled, sulfur dioxide gases mixes with water in the interior lining of the tiny air sacks (alveoli) in your lungs as well as the ducts (bronchi and bronchioles) that deliver air to the lungs. When sulfur dioxide reacts with water, it forms sulfuric acid.

Sulfuric acid is one of the strongest acids known to science. It can damage delicate tissues of the respiratory tract. In addition, when inhaled, sulfuric acid paralyzes the cilia in the respiratory track for about 15 minutes. These are tiny cellular organelles found on the surface of the cells lining much of the respiratory system. These motile organelles' job is to remove crud that deposits in the air passageways and move it toward the oral cavity. Here it can be swallowed or spit out. Paralyzing your cilia makes it impossible for the lungs to remove particulates you inhale. Particulates come from cigarette smoke, even secondary smoke, air pollution, marijuana, or smoke from fires. These particulates which can settle in the lung when cilia are incapacitated are often attached to heavy metals that could lead to lung cancer.

As if that's not bad enough, in the small air sacs in your lungs (the alveoli), sulfuric acid destroys their ultrathin walls. This causes the alveoli to break down. As they break down, the surface area for oxygen absorption decreases. This leads to emphysema. As more and more alveolar walls disintegrate, breathing becomes very difficult. This can lead to congestive heart failure.

That's not the only reason not to smoke Kratom or anything else. Anytime combustion occurs, for example, in a cigarette, nitrogen in the air, reacts with oxygen in the air to form nitrogen oxide gases. They combine with water in the respiratory system to create nitric acid, another super strong acid that can damage the delicate lining of the lungs.

Can Kratom leaves be chewed?

Freshly picked Kratom leaves can be chewed, but you might want to strip out the central vein of the plant. And be prepared for the potentially awful taste.

Once you've taken the leaf into your mouth, your job is to macerate or pulverize the leaf by chewing on it, like a cow chewing on its cud. When chewed up, swallow the stuff. You can chase it with water or a sweet liquid like OJ to rid the taste.

How many leaves should you chew at a time?

Some sources say chewing two or three is enough, although, you'll have to find out for yourself. Frankly we've both tried chewing green leaves from our Kratom plants growing in our Chinese greenhouse, and would not do it again -- ever!

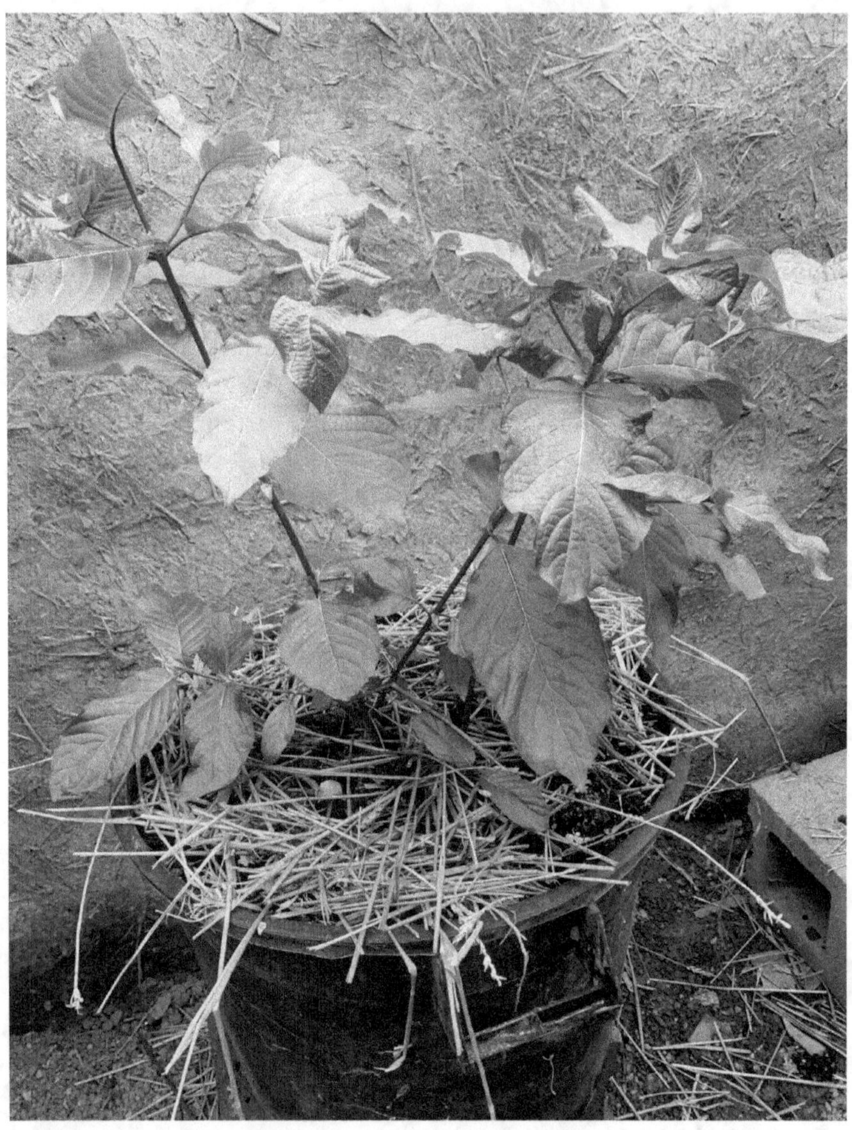

Kratom plant growing in our Chinese Greenhouse. We try to adjust our highly alkaline soil to an acidic pH between pH 5.5 and 6.5 by adding elemental sulfur. We also apply pH neutral water from our aquaponics system.

Kratom grows indoors well in moist, acidic soil. We also mulch our soils to help keep the soil moist and keep leaves from wilting.

SAFETY ISSUES

How long does it take to feel the effect?

Some people claim that they feel Kratom's effect within 10 to 15 minutes of ingestion. Others say it take a little longer – around 20 to 30 minutes. Still others say, Kratom effects are not felt for up to 40 minutes. Why's this?

As you learned earlier, how you ingest Kratom will greatly affect the speed with which the benefits start manifesting themselves. When ingested in a liquid like tea or chocolate almond milk, you'll very like feel the effect relatively quickly. If you're taking Kratom as a capsule, it could a bit take longer to begin feeling its effects. But even then, the speed with which the benefits are delivered may vary with the time of day, your state of mind, whether you're taking it on an empty stomach or after a big meal.

Bottom line: You'll have to find out for yourself.

We find that the effects manifest themselves very quickly but subtly. In other words, they slowly creep in.

How long do its benefits last?

Most people say that the effects of Kratom last 4 or 5 hours. Maybe up to six hours. We've found that 4 to 5 hours to be about right.

Is there a let-down like when coming off alcohol?

I (Dan) used to drink beer and wine, but as I got older found myself get extremely groggy after the alcohol buzz faded. I'd feel miserable for a couple hours.

Both Linda and I have found that Kratom's effects wear away gradually, almost imperceptibly. When they've worn off, we're left feeling well -- not tired or depressed like after alcohol. How you respond, of course, may differ.

IS KRATOM SAFE TO USE?

That's the million-dollar question.

People have been using Kratom for centuries with, as far as we can tell, little adverse side effect. That said, there are some cities, counties, and states in the US and some countries that have banned Kratom. In the US, a handful of states have pigeonholed Kratom in the category of Schedule 1 drugs. That infamous group includes some pretty dangerous drugs, notably morphine and cocaine and a not so dangerous herb, notably marijuana. The FDA and a number of other states are currently trying to figure out how to classify and regulate Kratom.

Schedule 1 drugs can be addictive. And, they are said to have no proven medical benefits. It's doubtful that this is true about Kratom, say proponents, including some rather distinguished researchers.

If you search the Internet, you will find that some people have died after ingesting Kratom. However, it appears that in virtually all of those cases Kratom was not the primary ingestible. Put another way, the people who died were taking another legal or illegal and potentially very dangerous drug, like heroin. They added Kratom to a mix of toxic chemicals circulating in their blood vessels and paid the price.

Researchers and advocates of Kratom use, like the American Kratom Association, point out that it's possible that the Kratom taken by some of these individuals could have been laced – either knowingly or unknowingly – with toxic drugs like hydrocodone.

Can Kratom be contaminated with potentially harmful bacteria?

In 2018, the FDA and the CDC (Centers for Disease Control) launched an investigation into an outbreak of salmonella infections thought to be caused by certain Kratom-containing products.

The found that 199 people had become sick in 41 states by the salmonella contaminated Kratom products. While problematic, it's probably not a good reason to ban them. Similar outbreaks have occurred with vegetables like lettuce and tomatoes.

All in all, it appears as if Kratom is pretty safe to use. But don't take our word. Research this topic fully.

Is Kratom addictive?

Opinions vary.

Some people assert that Kratom is addictive. Others say "No, not at all." Still others say, "Yeah, maybe psychologically addictive...like coffee."

By and large, most sources say people can become dependent

on Kratom, even addicted to it, but the addiction is pretty mild. Moreover, it's an addiction that can be cured pretty easily, they say.

Professor Walter Prozialeck, who teaches pharmacology at Midwestern University, reviewed 100 scientific papers on Kratom's safety. In his review, published in 2016, he noted "By any measure, Kratom would be less harmful and less addictive than something like heroin. If you look at the evidence, you have to conclude that. But Kratom can induce a state of physical dependence." What's physical dependence?

According to the National Institute on Drug Abuse, a group within the US government's National Institutes of Health, physical dependence is a **physical condition caused by chronic use of a tolerance-forming drug, in which abrupt or gradual drug withdrawal causes unpleasant physical symptoms.**

Physical dependence is a fairly common problem that may occur with the chronic use of many drugs, even low-dose prescription drugs taken as instructed. Physical dependence can develop from low-dose therapeutic use of certain medications such as benzodiazepines, opioids, antiepileptics and antidepressants, as well as recreational drugs such as alcohol, opioids, amphetamines, and benzodiazepines.

If Professor Prozialeck is right, Kratom is less addictive than dangerous drugs like heroin, but could induce physical dependence, meaning you will have an adverse physical reaction to Kratom if you stop taking it.

What's the difference between physical dependence and addiction?

According to the NIDA, "physical dependence in and of itself does not constitute addiction..." Addiction is the compulsive use of a drug. Individuals who are addicted to a drug are unable to stop using it. Moreover, drug use may cause them to falter socially. They often fail to do what they're supposed to do at work and at home. They may shirk family obligations and not show up to work at all. In addition, addicts suffer from withdrawal. Withdrawal symptoms may be physical or mental and can be quite severe.

So, are they splitting hairs here? The experts say that a person can become physically dependent on drugs, such as pain meds. They may develop a tolerance to the drug, meaning they have to take more and more to get the relief they need. The line between physical dependence and addiction though is this: If they cannot live without the drug, they're addicted.

How can Kratom addictions be treated?

Kratom may be psychologically addictive like almost anything, even coffee, chocolate and sex. It may be physically addictive. That's the bad news.

The good news, say several authors, is that if you take Kratom infrequently, and regularly switch from red to green to white, your chances of becoming addicted may be greatly reduced.

In other good news, the addiction is pretty easy to kick and withdrawal symptoms are, reportedly, rather mild compared to those experienced when coming off wicked drugs like heroin and morphine.

Professor Christopher McCurdy, who teaches medicinal chemistry at the University of Florida says that Kratom "...is probably addictive, but it's addictive equivalent is something like coffee..." (You'll recall that Kratom is in the coffee tree family.)

By all means, read the books available through Barns and Noble or Amazon in which authors describe their addiction to Kratom. If you have an addictive personality, you may want to seriously consider not taking Kratom.

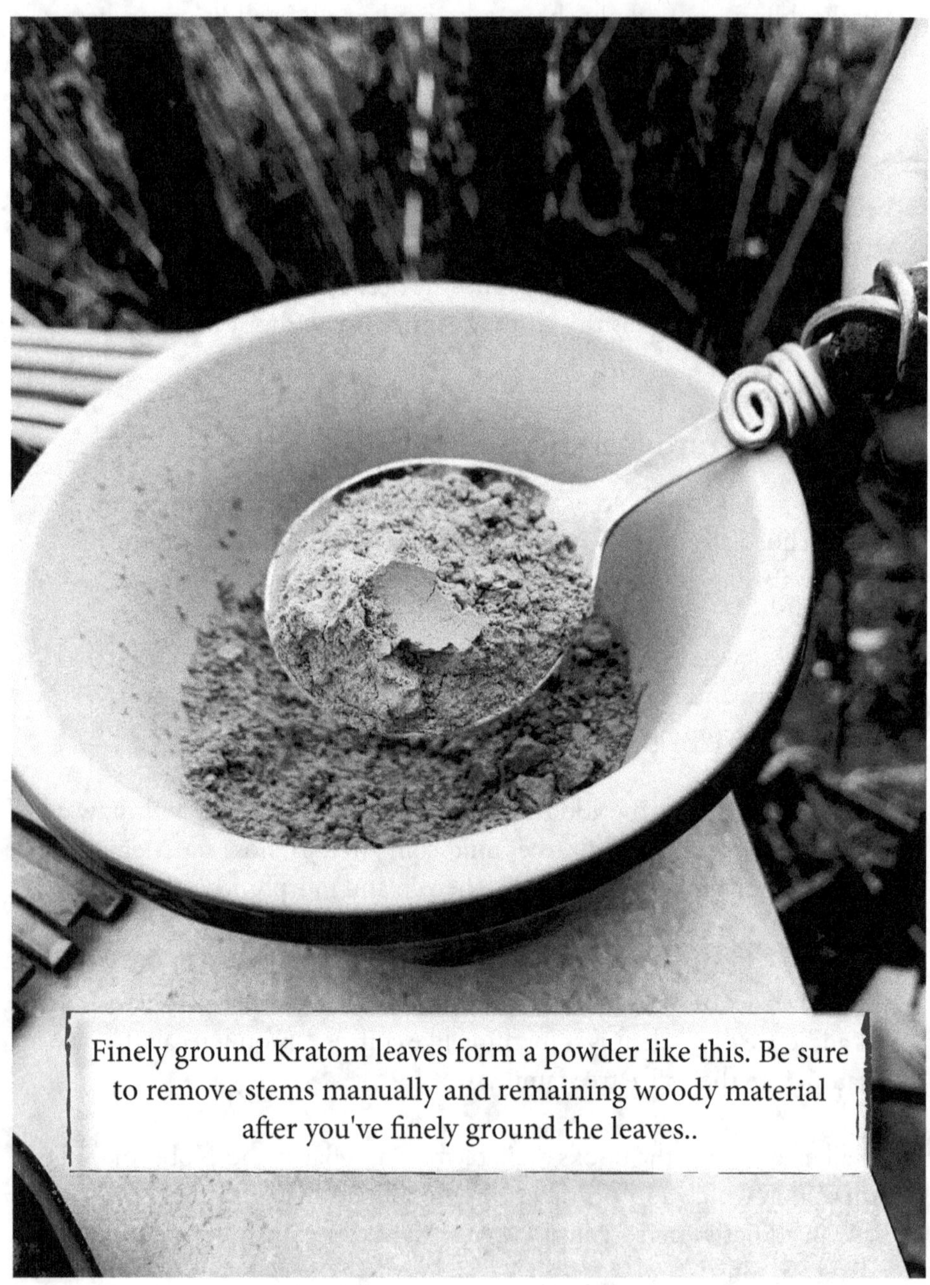

Finely ground Kratom leaves form a powder like this. Be sure to remove stems manually and remaining woody material after you've finely ground the leaves..

10

WHERE CAN I LEARN MORE ABOUT KRATOM?

Are there any books on Kratom you should read?

Although we've tried to write a fairly comprehensive book, it's always a good idea to read as much as you can about a subject. We were surprised to find numerous books in paperback and electronic format on Kratom on the Internet. We also were surprised to find that most of the books are rather tiny tomes, hardly worth calling "books." Booklets might be a more appropriate term. We even found that a few authors padded their books – for instance, used larger font size and extra space between lines – to make a tiny bit of information appear worthy of booklet status.

Padding was a trick Dan's college students used to employ on term papers. To satisfy the 10-page requirement, they'd often expand margins, increase the font size, and, when desperate, switch to triple spacing, assuming he was too stupid to figure out their subterfuge.

(After a few years of teaching, he switched to a word-count rather than a page-count requirement.)

The brevity of these books means that most of them are pretty superficial. As we started reading the books, we also found that a few of them were rather poorly written. Moreover, most are written by biased advocates of Kratom use.

Are there any good books on Kratom?

Dan's read eight books on Kratom. Here are the ones he thinks are the most readable, reliable, accurate, and hence useful.

So far, there are four books I'd pass on to someone and say, "Here, read this. It's pretty reliable and well written."

The first book is Kratom self-published by Paul White. It has a massive subtitle: *Everything you need to know about Kratom powder (extract, capsules, herbal supplement) for pain management: it's uses, benefits, possible side effects, dosage and interactions.* All in all, it does a pretty good job. The only mistake I found is in the way the author classifies Kratom trees by vein color, which is a common mistake virtually all the books make.

The second book is *CBD vs Kratom: Your Ultimate Guide to Understand CBD Oil and Kratom* by Frank Coles. This is the best book I've encountered. It is full of good information on ways to take Kratom, notably how to make pastes, teas, etc. – although I've covered the subject in great deal, Frank Coles provides exact recipes. Coles recommends doses, although, I'd take his recommendations as rough guidelines and always start with low doses to see how you are affected. Be sure to keep records, pay attention to your physiological and mental state to judge your response.

The third book I'd recommend is *Kratom Addiction* by Jerry Foster and Darnell Denton, the former who says he knows how to prevent

Kratom addiction, the latter who says he was addicted to it. This book, like some of the others comes with a paragraph-long subtitle: ***Everything you need to know about Kratom: How You can prevent and treat Kratom tolerance, abuse, and addiction (Kratom for beginners, Cure for Pain, Anxiety, Stress, and Addiction).*** It's worth reading to learn about the potential for and cure of Kratom addiction. It's best to go into these things with eyes and minds wide open.

The fourth book ***Kratom: The Complete Introduction for Beginners with Everything you Need to Know About Kratom!*** It's quite well written and appears to be rather scientifically sound.

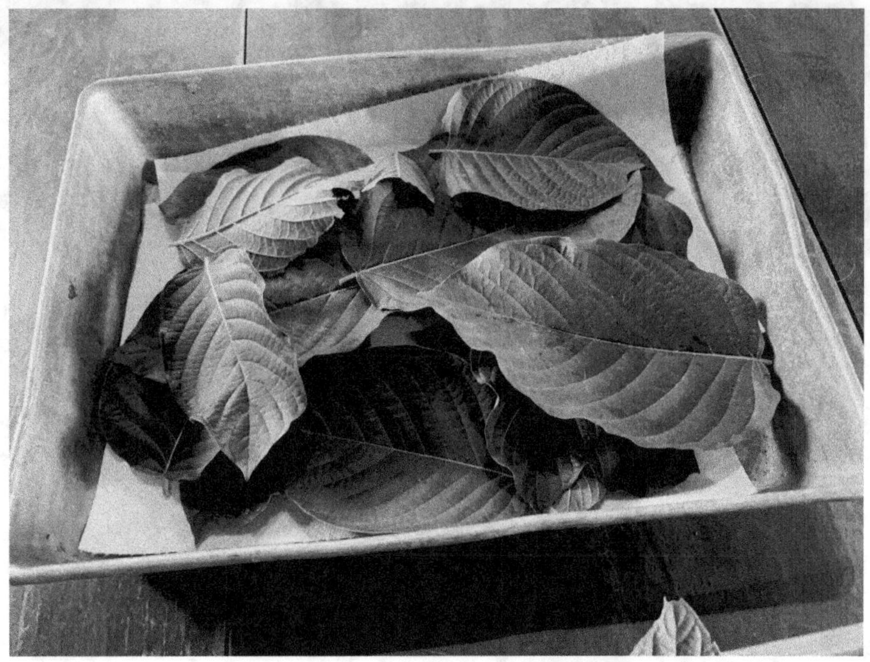

Kratom leaves from Dan and Linda's plants being dried on our kitchen table in a baking pan to make tea leaves and powder.

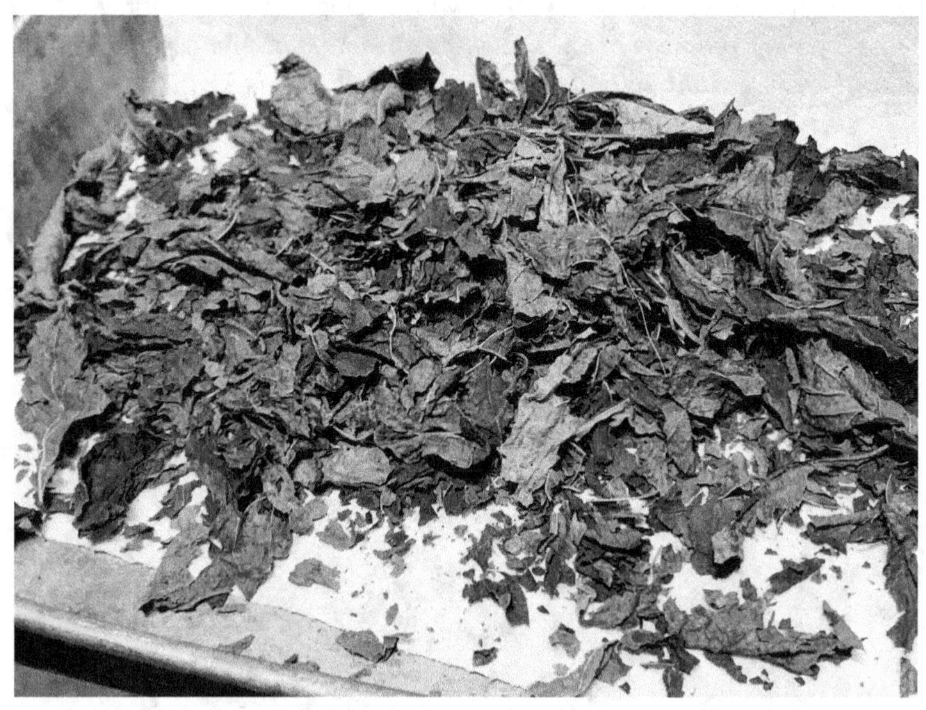

Two days later we were able to crush the leaves into much smaller pieces. In a couple more days, we will grind them up a bit more to make tea leaves we can place in a tea strainer.

11

CAN YOU GROW KRATOM AND MAKE YOUR OWN POWDER?

Can Kratom be grown in areas outside SE Asia?

Absolutely. If you live in a tropical climate, in a country like Costa Rica or Panama, for example, or in subtropical climate, like southern Florida, you can probably grow Kratom outdoors, year-round – so long as it is legal.

If you live further north, but still experience pretty warm weather year-round, you may be able to grow Kratom outdoors in the late spring, summer, and early fall. If temperatures drop below 50°F, however, you'll want to grow Kratom in pots outdoors, then move your plants indoors when temperatures start to drop. We have just started doing this.

Be careful when growing plants in pots, however. The soil in potted plants growing outdoors can dry out pretty quickly. Be sure to check the soil moisture level every day or two. Don't overwater. Waterlogging the roots, literally suffocates them. That's because water fills the air spaces in the soil and prevents roots from absorbing oxygen from the air that occupies the spaces between soil particles. Overwatering and underwater stresses plants and can kill them.

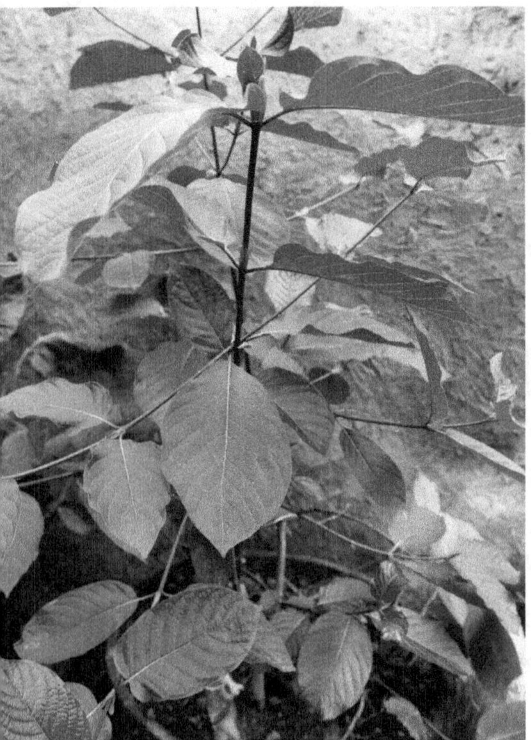

Can Kratom be grown indoors?

Yes, absolutely.

In colder climates, you can grow Kratom indoors or in heated greenhouses. Kratom can also be grown in homes and apartments near a sunny window or under grow lights. In the winter, when growing indoors, you will need to place your plants near a south-facing window. In the summer, you will very likely have to place them near an east- or west-facing window or haul them out to a sunny porch or sunny section of your back yard.

Can Kratom be grown in greenhouses?

Kratom can be grown in greenhouses year-round. Growing in greenhouses is a challenge. In colder climates, for example, year-round growing will require a source of heat for late fall, winter, and early spring. In the summer, greenhouses in most locations will also require some economical cooling system to maintain temperatures below 85°F. Shade cloth and fans may be required. Kratom likes temperatures in the 70s and 80s.

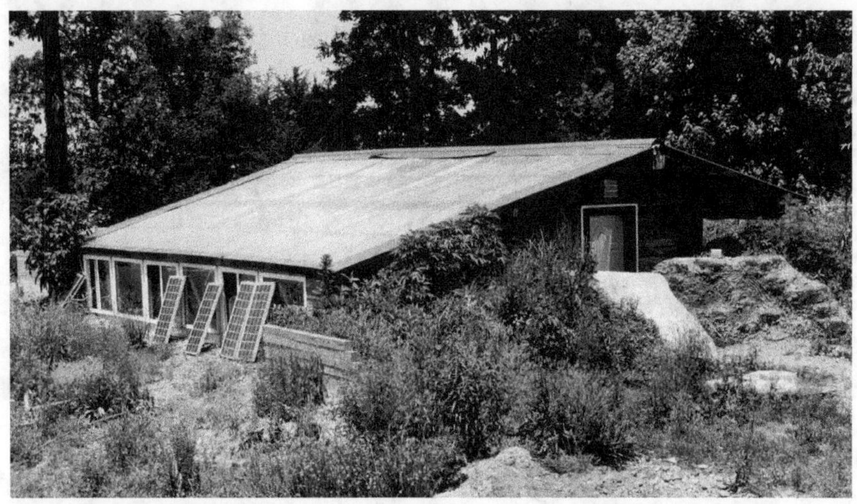

Heating and cooling can be quite expensive. To avoid this cost, we built a Chinese greenhouse. Chinese greenhouses are earth-sheltered greenhouses designed to allow one to grow warm weather plants year-round only using solar energy. They are a great alternative to an ordinary glass greenhouse or plastic hoop house.

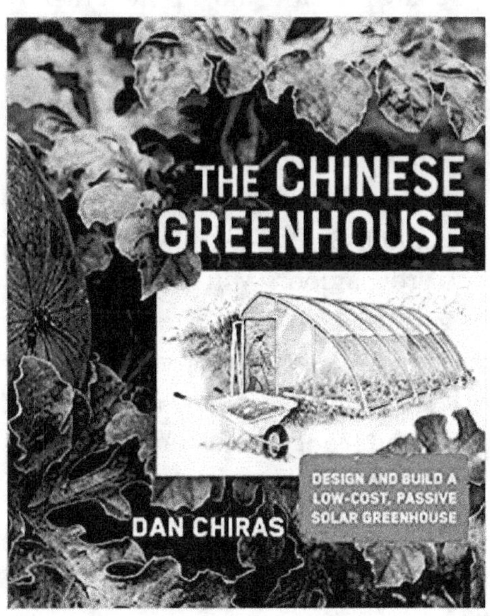

To learn more about Chinese greenhouses, you might want to read my book, *The Chinese Greenhouse*. You can purchase it through Barns and Noble, my publisher New Society, amazon, or through my website windrivermusic.net.

What special conditions are required for Kratom to grow well?

Kratom is a tropical plant, which means it likes warm temperatures – day and night -- and fairly high levels of humidity. As just noted, Indoor and outdoor temperatures in the 70s and 80s are ideal, but the plant can tolerate temperatures in the 90s. It can also tolerate colder temperatures -- down to around 50°F. Although cooler temperatures will slow the growth of the plant, they won't kill it.

Temperatures below 50°F, however can be problematic. Temperatures between 50°F and 32°F may not kill trees, but they will very likely cause them to lose their leaves. But don't worry, when temperatures warm up again, the leaves will very likely come back -- just as long as the plant hasn't frozen. If temperatures drop below freezing, your trees will very likely perish.

Warmth is not only essential for plant growth it increases the concentration of beneficial phytochemicals in the leaves. Leaves from plants grown in warmer temperatures are therefore more potent than leaves from Kratom trees grown in colder temperatures.

The lesson here is two-fold. Keep your plants warm year round, or, if that's not possible, harvest leaves primarily during warmer weather.

Kratom likes high humidity too. Greenhouses tend to be fairly humid. Homes tend to be less humid. If you grow indoors, you may want to mist your plants two or three times a day. Bear in mind, though, that too much humidity can result in the buildup of mold and mildew on leaves. If growing in a greenhouse, I'd recommend keeping a fan on your plants to promote air circulation and reduce mold and mildew.

What kind of soil should you use?

Kratom grows in tropical soils which are, contrary to popular belief, rather nutrient poor. The tropical rainforest is a paradox. It's the most diverse and abundant terrestrial biome on planet Earth, but it springs from the poorest of soils. In fact, when tropical rainforests are cleared and the land is planted in crops, soil nutrients are typically used up within a few years, so much so that crops begin to fail.

The reason abysmally poor tropical rain forest soils support its luxuriant plant community is that plant nutrients are very rapidly recycled in these ecosystems. Leaves or branches of trees and other forms of vegetation that drop to the ground, quickly decompose. They are broken down by insects and a whole host of microbes – bacteria and fungi. Biological decay releases the nutrients in decaying plant matter back into the soil where they are quickly taken up by the roots of tropical plants.

In a tropical rainforest, then, most of the nutrients in this ecosystem are plant bound. As long as the nutrient recycling continues, though, plants thrive. Removing that mass of nutrients – the trees and other vegetation – disrupts the rain forests active nutrient cycles. It eliminates the leaves and branches that fall to replenish the soil. As a result, tropical rainforests can become quite barren, rather quickly.

So, what kind of soil should you use? Will a nutrient-poor soil work?

When growing Kratom in soil, either outdoors in your backyard or in pots in a greenhouse or your home, the best results occur when using an organic-rich container soil. I used to make my own mixes from native soil, composted manure, and other organic matter. I have much better luck using a commercial product, Miracle Gro's Container Mix.

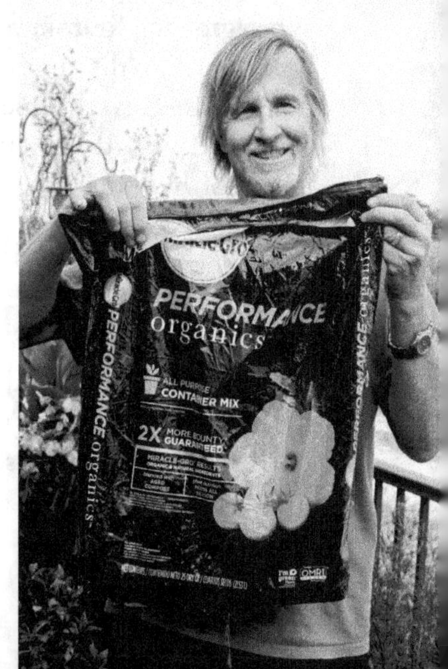

How do you prevent Kratom from growing into a tree?

If you want to grow Kratom indoors in a greenhouse or near a south-facing window in your home, you must prevent the tiny seedling you buy (a well-rooted cutting) from developing into a 50-foot tall tree, that pokes holes in your roof.

This can be achieved by planting Kratom in smaller pots – for example, 3-to-5 gallon pots – and by pruning the branches several times each year. Both practices will limit growth.

Pruning Kratom is much like pruning bushes growing in a yard. Snip off the ends of branches and cut off the main vertical stem. These measures will help create bush-like plants rather than tall unruly trees.

Do you need artificial lighting when growing in a greenhouse?

Being tropical, Kratom plants like lots of sunlight. They'll survive in as few as five hours of light a day, or so we're told, but thrive when exposed to much longer photoperiods (periods of sunlight).

When growing Kratom year-round in a greenhouse, Kratom plants will be subjected to the same daylight schedule Mother Nature imposes on us humans. This schedule varies depending on your latitude. In the equator, daylength is pretty much the same all year round, but as you move north or south from the equator, daylight shifts. Summers offer many hours of sunshine and fewer hours of darkness. Winter offers just the opposite.

To enhance plant growth in the fall, winter, and spring in a greenhouse, you may want to suspend grow lights over your plants to promote the best growth. I highly recommend LED grow lights over all other types, in large part because they are energy efficient. I also highly recommend grow lights sold by Happy Leaf (happyleaf.com). They are durable, relatively inexpensive, energy-efficient, and more importantly produce just the right light plants need to grow. Unlike most other lights used for growing plants, Happy Leaf LED grow lights generate about 65% red light, 15% blue light, and 20% green light, which is the photosynthetically active radiation on which plants do best. (More on this shortly.)

Do you need artificial lighting when growing in your home?

You can grow indoors near a window, but the amount of light entering your home or apartment varies by season. In northern temperate climates, which includes most of the United States, you'll find that south-facing windows provide the most sunshine in the winter. That's because, the Sun carves a very low path across the sky in the winter, and therefore shines into your home through south-facing glass.

In the summer, plants placed in or near south-facing windows will receive very little sunlight. That's because the summer sun cuts a very high path across the sky. Sunlight beats down on the roof of your home but doesn't enter south-facing windows most of the summer, if your home is equipped with eaves or overhangs.

In this case, you should move your Kratom plants to east- or west-facing windows in the summer or provide additional lighting at the end of each day with a timer-controlled LED grow light. Or, you can move the plants outdoors.

What kind of Grow light should you use?

Plants love sunlight. As you may know, sunlight appears white, but is actually made up of a rainbow of colors: red, orange, yellow, green, blue, and violet light. Each has its own wavelength. Interestingly, plants selectively absorb mostly red and blue light. It's these wavelengths that power photosynthesis. They make up the photosynthetically active radiation (PAR).

Good grow lights that provide mostly red, blue, and green wavelength light are ideal for growing plants like Kratom. But not all grow lights are created equal. Cheaper LED grow lights may contain more red and blue light, but not in the right proportion. Studies carried out at Purdue University show that the grow lights that promote the optimum growth contain PAR that is 65% red light, 15% blue light, and 20% green light. That's shown in the graph below.

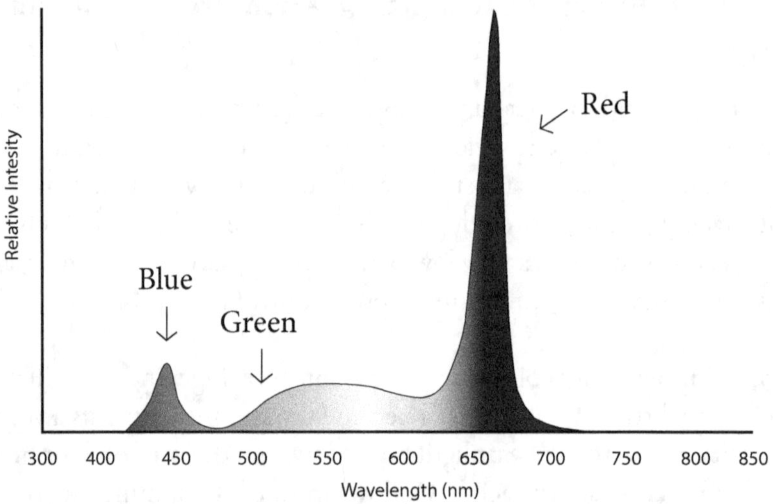

Unfortunately, there aren't many grow lights – LED or otherwise – that achieve this goal. Check out the wavelengths produced by a standard fluorescent light bulb.

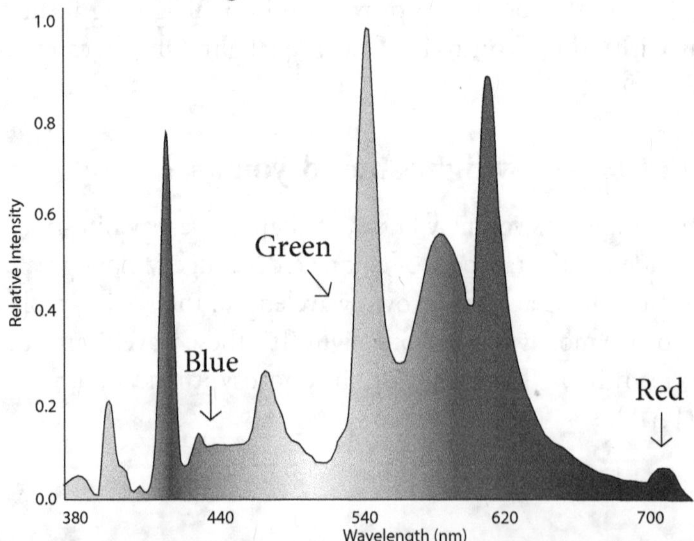

I've found that Happy Leaf's lights match plants' requirements for red, blue, and green light, which is why we use them in our greenhouse. Below is a photo of some leafy greens growing in my basement under LED lights that I purchased from Happy Leaf.

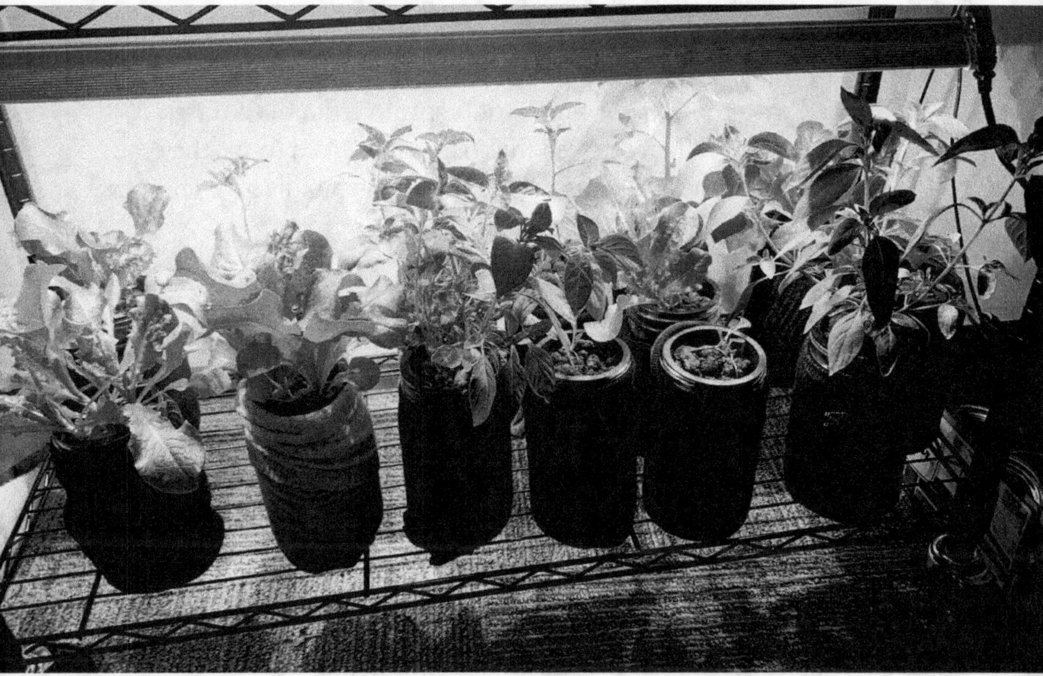

We've found that grow lights also vary with respect to quality. There are some enticingly inexpensive LED grow lights on the market, but the cheapest lights are invariably made from inexpensive materials like plastic, provide much less PAR than you need, and may not last as long as well-made and more expensive lights. You truly get what you pay for. So whatever you do, don't shop by price.

How do you grow Kratom?

Kratom can be grown from seeds or cuttings.

Kratom seeds can be purchased online, but we don't recommend this route. Growers find it extremely difficult to get Kratom seeds to germinate. According to mytreesoflife.com, a supplier of high-quality cuttings, "Seeds rapidly degrade after being released from the plant, so germination rates decrease very quickly from that point on, and the seeds do not store well."

A far better option is to buy cuttings. Cuttings are just that: tiny end sections of branches that are placed in potting soil. If cut properly and treated with rooting hormone, roots sprout from the cut stem, creating seedlings. When the seedlings have established roots, they can be transplanted into larger pots, where they grow rapidly given proper temperature, light, humidity, and soil pH.

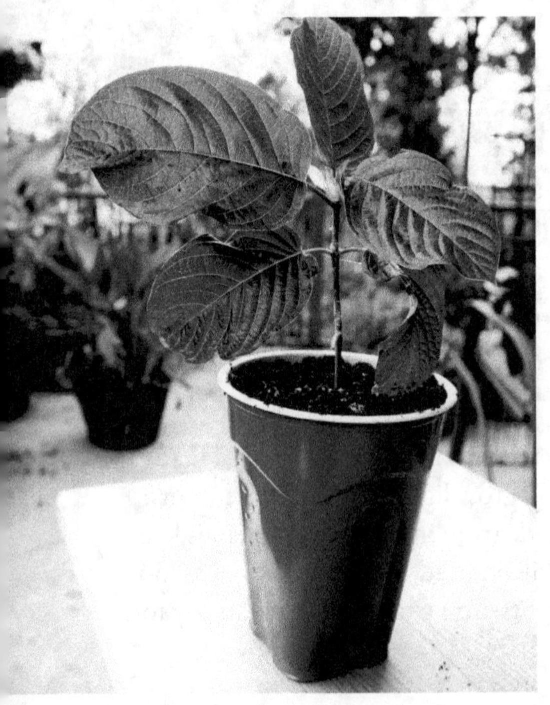

Here's a seedling I purchased from mytreesoflife.com.

It's now a healthy 6 foot tall bush growing in my greenhouse.

We started harvesting leaves from this plant within 6 months

When Can Your Harvest Leaves?

The leaves of the Kratom tree can grow quite large – up to 7 inches long and 4 inches wide. In the wild, leaf production is greatest in the wet season. In dry periods, the trees often drop their leaves to reduce the tree's water demands and help it survive.

When growing your own, indoors or outdoors, it is best to harvest leaves in warmer periods. That's because the leaves contain more beneficial phytochemicals at such times.

When growing your own trees from seeds, we're told that it can take up to take to two years before leaves are mature and are producing the right stuff – alkaloids and other phytochemicals. When growing from cuttings, leaves can be harvested much more quickly, even when the plants are only a few feet tall because cuttings are taken from already mature trees.

How do you dry Kratom leaves?

Kratom leaves can be dried in a small electric dehydrator like the one shown in the photo below. We've found that this is the easiest way to dry small quantities of leaves. Using this method, leaves dry quickly, within a day or so, becoming quite crisp and crumbly like dry autumn leaves. Dried leaves can then be slightly crushed to produce tea leaves or ground further into a powder.

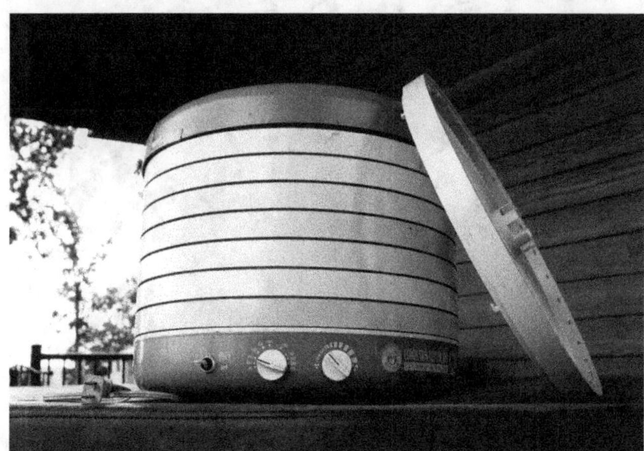

Large quantities of leaves can also be dried on clean metal or plastic screens – like window screens – for those of us living in more arid climates or during dryer periods for those of us living in more humid environments. Spread them thin so leaves do not pile on top of one another. Overlapping may retard drying and may promote mold growth, ruining part of your harvest.

If you purchase plants, consult with your supplier on the best way to dry the leaves. Ask him or her whether they should be dried in sunlight or under artificial light – or some combination of the two -- or no light at all.

How do you make powder from Kratom leaves?

Leaves can be ground in a coffee grinder or a kitchen blender. Creating a fine powder could take up to five minutes. When done, store the powder into plastic bags or, better yet, glass jars and seal them tight.

Leaves can also be ground by hand using a mortar and pestle, as shown in the figure below. **No matter how you grind your leaves, be sure to remove stems and the central vein of leaves before you grind them up. This will yield a finer powder.**

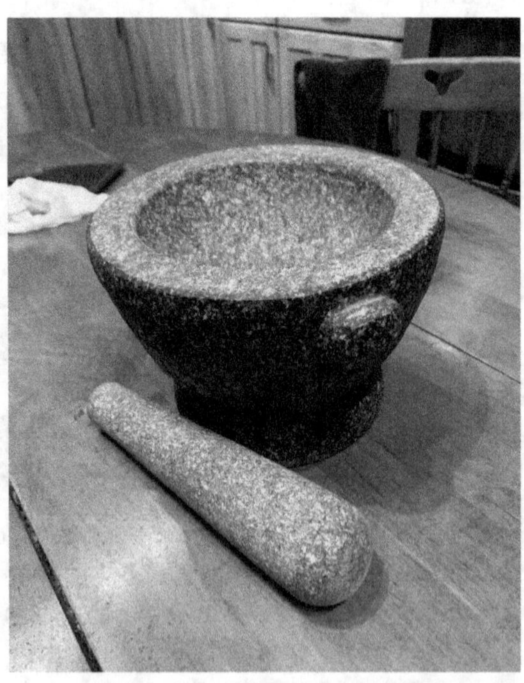

12

LEGAL ISSUES

What's Kratom's legal status in the US and abroad?

Kratom's legal status varies throughout the world and even within countries. In some countries Kratom is illegal. That is to say, it is illegal to possess, sell, use, and grow Kratom. I'll tell you which ones fall into this category shortly.

In other countries, Kratom is legal but only with a doctor's prescription.

In the vast majority of nations, however, Kratom is unregulated. Most people take that to mean that it is legal.

Let's begin by looking at Kratom's legal status in the United States.

Is Kratom Legal in the United States?

Kratom's legal status is a mixed bag in the States. Although it is not federally regulated, at least for now, **Kratom has been made illegal in:**

- Wisconsin
- Vermont
- Rhode Island
- Indiana
- Arkansas
- Alabama

Kratom is illegal in multiple cities and counties across the states as well as on all US military bases. This list is ever changing as more legislation is passed and updated. For an up to date list we encourage you to do your own research. Check out the Kratom legality map at the following website: Kraoma.com

What does it mean when we say that Kratom is unregulated?

Kratom's unregulated status means that the US government, in particular the Food and Drug Administration, has not issued any restrictions on the sale, possession, or use of Kratom. Presumably it is legal to grow, too.

Although this description seems pretty cut and dry, it's not. Why?

Even though, Kratom may be legal to grow it, sell, and use it in much of the US, it's not legal to import Kratom into the country. Imported Kratom is subject to seizure by the Feds, although that hasn't seemed to stop its importation.

Is the US Government Going to Ban Kratom?

On August 31, 2016, the U.S Drug Enforcement Administration (DEA) published a ruling temporarily listing mitragynine and 7-hydroxymitragynine, the main psychoactive constituents of Kratom, as Schedule I drugs. Labeling Kratom as a Schedule 1 drug places it in the same family as heroin, LSD, cocaine, Peyote, methamphetamines, marijuana, and Ecstasy. In case you don't know, a **schedule 1 drug is a potentially addictive drug and one that the FDA says has no medical value.**

The DEA's ruling led to widespread public furor. Thousands of Kratom users objected, arguing that the DEA did not have the data to make such a determination. In addition, many individuals pointed out that the DEA was ignoring the reported benefits and was exaggerating or misinterpreting reports on addiction and side effects. This uproar, in turn, caused the agency to withdraw its recommendation two months later. Since then, the DEA has been reviewing studies and testimony from individuals and various organizations to determine if any action should be taken—specifically, how Kratom's major ingredients should be classified.

The future of Kratom in the US remains in limbo. To keep up to date on its legal status, be sure to log on to the American Kratom Association's web site. They keep close tabs on legal issues at all levels—local, state, federal. You might even want to join the organization to help them out.

With this information in mind, let's take a look at Kratom's status throughout the world, looking first to the United States' northern neighbor.

Is Kratom Legal in Canada?

Kratom is illegal in Canada, although you can burn Kratom incense (we're not sure why anyone would want to). Burn it, but don't consume it. And don't sell it. All this means is that Kratom is pretty much illegal in Canada.

Is Kratom Legal in Europe?

Kratom is illegal in most European countries, including Ireland, the United Kingdom, Sweden, Latvia, Lithuania, Denmark (really guys?), Romania, Poland, Hungary, Russia, and Italy. Kratom's use is regulated in one country: Finland. There it can only be used by individuals who have a doctor's prescription. There is a catch, however, it's illegal to import Kratom into Finland. In all other European countries, Kratom is currently unregulated.

Is Kratom Legal in Australia and New Zealand?

In Australia, Kratom is classified as a narcotic by the government. Their decision is said to be based on at least two factors: (1) it's being banned in countries where it grows and, incidentally, has been consumed for hundreds of years with very few problems, and (2) a study performed by Smith Cline, a major pharmaceutical company. We can rest assured that their report was unbiased.

In New Zealand, residents can purchase and use Kratom so long as they have a prescription from a doctor. If you don't have a prescription, it's a crime to possess and use it.

Is it legal in Southeast Asia and Surrounding areas?

Ironically, Kratom is illegal in several Southeast Asian countries. These include Thailand, Myanmar (formerly Burma), South Korea, and Malaysia. Heavy fines are levied against South Koreans and Malaysians caught using or selling Kratom. In Malaysia, you may be given a long jail sentence, up to four years.

So what' the deal with Thailand where Kratom has been used for decades and also grows in the wild?

On the surface, Thailand's ban on Kratom seems like a paradox. When you uncover the facts, though, you see that it's just another government action with less-than-admirable motives. Here's the story:

As many readers know, opium has been widely used in the tiny nation of Thailand for many years. What many don't know is that the government regulated and taxed its sale. In addition, taxes generated rather sizeable revenues for the Thai government.

In 1943, government banned Kratom. Why?

The government knew that Kratom grew wild which made it relatively inexpensive. Its local availability and low price meant that many people were using Kratom instead of opium whose sale was generously taxed.

At that point in Thailand's history, the Thai government badly needed money to wage a war, the East Asian War, which had broken out the previous year. The government had two choices: they could regulate and tax Kratom to raise money or ban it outright so more people would theoretically return to opium, which would help fund the war. Not surprisingly, they chose the latter. Besides, who would want to tax a substance that was so inexpensive, even free, because it grew wild in parts of Thailand?

On January 7, 1943 Police Major General Pin Amornwisaisoradej (that's a tongue twister!), who was also a member of Thailand's House of Representative, summed it up like this: "Taxes for opium are high while Kratom is currently not being taxed. With the increase of those taxes, people are starting to use Kratom instead and this has had a visible impact on our government's income."

Hence the ban. If convicted of possession and or use, Thai people could spend up to one year in jail. If convicted of more serious crimes of producing, importing, exporting, selling, possessing Kratom with intent to sell, they can be incarcerated for up to 2 years. Fortunately, people arrested for Kratom-related offenses rarely go to jail.

Kratom remains illegal in Thailand today, despite efforts to change its status. Not surprisingly, opium use continues to rise. There is hope among Thai citizens that Kratom will someday be decriminalized.

Should Kratom be banned or regulated?

Many individuals believe that Kratom should not be banned but should be regulated. Some individuals and organizations call for regulations on products – powder, pills, etc. – **to ensure that consumers end up with a pure product, unadulterated by potentially harmful chemicals or laced with useless chemical fillers** – a problem that's currently encountered in the CBD market.

Supporters of Kratom regulations also argue that it is imperative that companies prepare their products safely so there is no chance of bacterial contamination, a rare but possible outcome, and that they test products, **so consumers know their purity and potency.**

Don't ban Kratom, they say, apply sensible regulations.

Should You Travel with Kratom?

Traveling with Kratom in your possession is inadvisable in states, cities, counties, or countries where Kratom is illegal. When traveling elsewhere, it's a good idea to be as inconspicuous as possible. You may want to place Kratom capsules in an empty herbal med container, for example, one that once contained Valerian Root, Passionflower, Golden seal, or Echinacea. We keep them in our suitcase, not in the glove compartment or console.

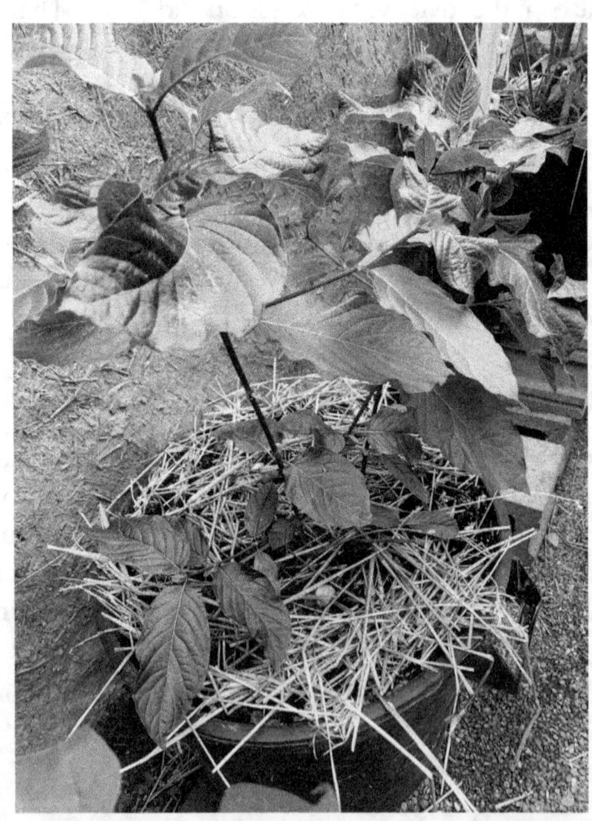

AFTERWORD

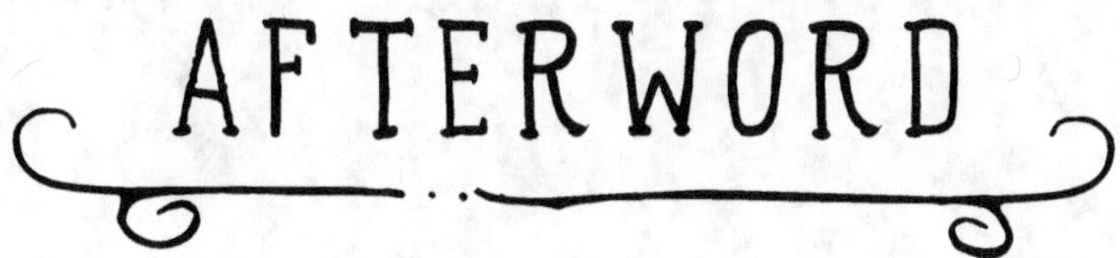

Hope you have enjoyed – and profited from – our little book. We've enjoyed studying the subject, assimilating this information, and writing up our findings.

At this point, there's not much more to say. From what we've seen and experienced, we think that Kratom -- like THC and CBD -- very likely offers some significant health benefits. It's not a miracle cure, by any means, but it does appear to offer wide-ranging mental and physical benefits. You need to make a decision on your own.

Our experience, though limited, has been quite positive. That said, we're keeping a careful eye out for further research by unbiased medical scientists on the benefits and side effects. We're intensely interested in research on topics such as drug interactions, tolerance, dependence, and addiction.

We'll also be carefully following the legal status of Kratom over the next few years. With the legalization of THC in many states -- for medical and recreational use -- and the widespread acceptance and use of CBD oil, we think the path for Kratom's legalization may be a bit easier. But who knows?

Be sensible, be careful, be mindful, and be well.